Lifting My Spirits

A Lifelong Dream Deferred No
Longer - Transformation from Fat
Chick to Bodybuilder After Age 50.

TAMMY WHITE

ISBN-13: 978-1725553439
ISBN-10:1725553430

For my mom, Betty.

It took me a few years to realize you taught me
everything I needed to know about how to be strong.
I am my mother's daughter.

And for Paula.

I needed to borrow some of your courage, my friend.

Contents

Disclaimer

This book is not intended as a substitute for the medical advice of physicians. The reader should regularly consult a physician in matters relating to his/her health and particularly with respect to any symptoms that may require diagnosis or medical attention.

Forward

Change.

How can one single word create so many different emotions in so many different people? Consider flashbacks to a time when an unexpected shift took place and you had to be innovative when you weren't quite ready to be. You survived the change, and in some cases grew from it. However, we still actively avoid change when possible.

As we get older, this seems to be more and more the case. We don't seek novelty, and we are less likely to take up challenges that make us feel unsure. Despite all the growth, we know that the other end of the journey is likely filled with conflict. Even when we know, without a doubt, that what we truly want is on the other side of said conflict. At best, we put it off and wait for the day when change is more convenient.

In my experience, the longer that we put it off, the more we continue to charge up the power that our fears have over us. The longer that we put it off, the less likely we are to step up to the challenge and enjoy the fruits of our labor.

Upon reflecting, this is the part about Tammy White's story that captivates me the most: the resistance that she had to overcome to create that initial inertia. I place myself in her shoes and allow myself to envision her mindset at that time. It takes life in my head. The fears, frustrations, and the many temptations to turn back to what was comfortable... oh what a challenge that must have been!

Her "before and after" pictures capture the accumulated glory, but I can't stare at them for long without thinking about all the obstacles that had to be overcome along the way.

The truth is Tammy sought guidance from me when the hardest work had already been done. She was looking to go from a "gym rat" that trained like a competitive athlete, to an actual competitive athlete. I didn't get the opportunity to live vicariously through her as she went toe to toe with the hardest leg of her fitness journey. The parts that I do know are solely through my educated imagination on these matters regarding what it takes to accomplish such a feat. That, and her almost always too modest recollection.

While working with Tammy, her new habits frequently and joyfully come to mind. This includes the modest and small details, such as explaining to me internet-world things that only millennials should know - to flat out doing a 180 with regards to her career and recently starting from scratch. Like all of us, she has fears. Unlike all of us, she is immediately able to weed out the irrational to keep her feet moving towards her goals. When I push her to uncomfortable places as an athlete, it's the exact same "poker face", and it's followed up by the most appropriate of actions.

While the physical transformation has been unbelievable, it's the abilities that came along with it that I find the most inspiring. If something in her world, something that disrupts her peace of mind, requires her to get up and do something about it... she just does. The old Nike marketing campaign comes to mind when I think of Tammy and her positive impact on my life. When something is not right, I think to myself, "You need to pull a Tammy."

"Just change it."

Alberto Nunez, 3D Muscle Journey

Introduction

One Sunday afternoon in March 2009, I was lying in a bed in an emergency room hooked up to machines monitoring my vitals. My husband was in a chair next to the bed, pale with worry as we waited for the doctor to come back with test results.

Four hours later, the doctor told us "you didn't have a cardiac event – this time. But it was smart to come in. A woman your age, in your condition…it was smart to come in." (I was 47 at the time.)

And then the other shoe dropped…

"If you don't change your life, you are likely to have a catastrophic cardiac event before you're 60."

I'm a wife and a busy teacher. After years of self-neglect, I found myself in an ER. And I *wasn't surprised* to hear that I was likely to die sooner rather than later.

What happened to me? Life happened.

Nothing notable about my life up to that point. Married, but not blessed with children, even though I wanted to be a mom since I was little. I compensated by throwing myself into teaching. I loved my job and said "yes" to too many things. Easily worked 50-60 hours a week. Some stress at home at times because my husband was married to a workaholic.

Each year I gained a little weight. That's normal, right? Still, I tried and quit several diet and exercise programs. Got busy, lost motivation, always thought I had time...sound familiar?

By age 46, I was on high blood pressure medication.

Fast forward a year - I was struggling daily with anxiety and sadness. I suspected I was having an anxiety attack that afternoon, but I asked my husband to drive me to the ER because the chest pains would not subside. My mother had died of a brain aneurysm, my father had triple by-pass surgery, and a grandfather died early of a heart attack. And that afternoon, I was worried that I had let my genetics catch up to me.

When the doctor told us that it was anxiety and not a heart attack, I did feel relieved. I could have just gone home and resumed life as usual. But something else happened. A switch flipped in my mind. I knew I was given a warning. I KNEW it. Something was different.

I could see the rest of my short life clearly from that day forward. I knew every tomorrow would be the same as every yesterday if I didn't change my life. I couldn't accept that. There was no more time to think about it. Every day that I didn't act was a day that I wouldn't get back. At that point, I promised myself that I would start and NOT quit. I promised that *this would be the last time I would start over*. There was no Plan B. ✳

Maybe that's a midlife crisis? I don't know. Midlife crisis or divine intervention? I'd like to think it's the latter.

I didn't quit. I'm writing this book to help you not quit.

I'm writing this book so that you will believe in your ability to prioritize self-care even when you feel guilty for using time and money to do it.

I'm writing this book for the people in your life that want those extra years with you.

I'm still a regular person and life never let up throwing curveballs. There have been tough times financially when the economy tanked in our state. There have been car accidents, illnesses, hospitalizations, broken appliances, job transfers, and Lord knows teaching never got easier.

The decision to become a bodybuilder in my fifties was a bit ballsy. I own that. In this book, I'll explain why it was important that I set that Big Scary Goal. There have been obstacles, setbacks, huge disappointments, and a challenging mental game I didn't expect.

But I didn't quit.

I've always quit before. I know my ER visit was upsetting, but plenty of people have experiences like that and still can't navigate the obstacles to change their lives. Some do. I'm grateful I was able to do it. And surprised considering my history of quitting. Why did it work this time? How did I do it?

Better question – are you ready to do it, too?

My hope is that this book will become your handbook for "how to not quit". I've organized the chapters so you can refer back to them in any order. When you read them in order, there will be some repetition of thoughts.

My story is in here, but so are my observations, some hard lessons, and some practical tips. I don't think most people quit because of some major event – they quit because life happens and old habits are hard to unlearn. I want to help you think of ways to organize your new life to make new habits. I want to help you change your mindset. I want to help you reach your goals.

At the end of each chapter, I've included a blank page for you to use for notes, thoughts, or questions you may have as you read.

If you find this book to be helpful or if you have questions, feel free to email me at <u>LiftingMySpirtitsBook@gmail.com</u> .

There are places in the book where I wanted to share my mindset at a specific point in time, so I borrowed posts from my own blog. My blog at <u>www.LiftingMySpirits.com</u> documents my entire journey since 2010.

Chapter 1

Can Damage from Self-Neglect Be Reversed?

"For nothing is impossible with God."
Luke 1: 37

"Only I can change my life.
No one can do it for me."
Carol Burnett

How many years of self-neglect can pass before we have medical problems that can't be reversed? I will share how I did exactly that in this chapter. But first, let me provide more details about how I got started, how I almost quit, and what kept me going.

A Self-Neglected Busy Teacher: 1997-2009

I was a busy high school teacher. Too many hours worked, high stress, bad eating habits, a little too many adult beverages, and sleep deprivation caught up to me. My mother died from a brain aneurysm when she was 56, so I knew I was at risk – but I always thought I had time. When I started gaining weight, I believed the "experts" who said that weight gain was something I should expect as I got older.

I joined a gym in 2006, but I didn't use it. Remember? Busy teacher. Busy and stressed.

When my doctor put me on blood pressure medication when I was in my mid-40's, I still didn't think that was due to anything other than "just getting older". So there I was – 47 years old, on high blood pressure meds, and my doctor was ready to start treating me for high cholesterol, too! I was at risk for several lifestyle-induced chronic illnesses.

March 2009: The ER Visit

One Sunday afternoon in March of 2009, sitting in the living room, I felt anxious, had a sharp pain in my chest, and I was dizzy.

"Honey – please take me to the ER."

When we arrived, I didn't have to wait long to be admitted, even though the waiting room was full. They, too, were concerned I was having a cardiac event. I was there for several hours, hooked up to machines, tests were run, all to get an idea of what was happening. My husband and I waited and hoped that all of it would rule out the worst.

The diagnosis? After four hours of tests and observation, the doctor said "it wasn't a cardiac event this time. It was an anxiety attack."

She emphasized the "this time". This young, female doctor pulled no punches. "A woman your age, in your physical condition… it was smart to come to the ER."

She went on to explain that *this time* it was not a cardiac event. But if I didn't change my life, I would have one before I was 60. I saw the blood drain out of my husband's face. I'm sure he saw the same when he looked at me.

I knew it. Deep down, I knew I was on borrowed time. My mother died young. She hadn't taken care of herself. She also let stress deteriorate the quality of her life. No one knows when their time is up, but this ER visit felt like a warning of things to come.

"Can't afford it" was one of my mental barriers to getting the help I needed to change my life. My copay for that ER visit was $1200. Add to that the monthly cost of blood pressure meds...add to that more meds that were on the horizon... it became obvious to me that money was going to be spent either way - treat a health problem <u>or prevent it</u>.

I can't remember exactly when it happened, but shortly after that ER visit, there was a moment when this thought hit me like an electric shock:

"You are God's kid and you're not taking care of yourself the way He expects you to."

Well, that put the guilt about the money and time spent on self-care into perspective in a heartbeat. I still struggled with it a bit out of habit, but my paradigm got shifted right at that moment. I didn't know exactly what I was going to do, but the decision was made. I was going to change.

I started walking. That's all I knew to do. I walked and researched my next move. I knew I needed help but didn't know what I needed or where to find it. So, all I did was walk. And I waited.

June 2009: Got a Gadget and Got Some Help

My school was out for summer vacation and I was at the gym in the middle of the day. I was walking on a treadmill on the second floor looking down at the central part of the gym. I saw a table of gadgets down by the front desk. On my way out, I stopped, pulled out a credit card, and left with one – a Bodybugg. For me, that was the corner that needed to be turned. I remember finally putting it together in my head...

"Let's throw some money at a solution. If I invest, I won't quit. I won't waste my money."

At that time, the Bodybugg company offered phone coaching, so I signed up for that, too. My phone coach was Kim. Her task was to teach me about the device and how to use the website interface, but what she really did was teach me how to eat and how to log what I ate. I listened. I implemented. I asked questions. I followed directions. I trusted. I did what I was told, and I got results. Who would have 'thunk' it?

Tracking provided data about food intake. The gadget provided an estimate of my calorie burn. Using that data daily to create a caloric deficit, I lost weight. Simple! Not easy to do, but a simple concept. Over the next nine months, I lost 40 pounds.

But...life happened. Progress stopped.

March 2010: Stalled

My Bodybugg coach had to quit coaching for personal reasons. Before she left, she made sure I was set up with knowledge and tools to continue. We both felt confident that I would be able to handle the things on my own. But there was a problem – my weight loss stopped. I also didn't see the results I wanted. I was lighter, yes, but I didn't look how I wanted to look. Something was missing. My weight started to increase and I didn't know why my cardio-only plan wasn't working anymore.

I joined a second gym - the local YMCA - hoping that a change of scenery would be helpful. I suspected that I needed to learn to how to weight train. Then, I did my research. What I suspected was true - I needed to learn how to lift to keep making progress. That's when I remembered my fascination with female bodybuilding back in the 1980's. I wanted to be a bodybuilder back then, but I was in my twenties and not a disciplined person. But older and wiser me thought, why not? *Why not?* Because I was scared. The idea of venturing into that part of the gym intimidated me. I wanted to do it, but I was afraid of looking stupid. And I was worried I would get hurt.

I tried to find a trainer who had experience teaching people my age how to lift. Met with a couple trainers, and both were friendly, but neither had the background knowledge I needed. Or if they did, they seemed more interested in helping me lower my expectations. Conversations were about how a woman "my age" should accept the situation and be realistic. I'm sure they meant well. It felt wrong, regardless. In hindsight, I used their response as an excuse to NOT learn how to lift because it scared me. I could have insisted. I didn't.

My insecure butt stayed on that treadmill. And my weight continued to creep up. The battle in my mind between wanting to learn to lift and the negative thoughts caused by insecurities, stopped me from getting off that safe treadmill. I was almost defeated by my own fears.

May 2010: Borrowed Courage

I reconnected with Paula on Facebook in 2010. Paula and I were friends in high school and had relocated to different states. To be perfectly honest, we weren't that close in high school. I thought she was reckless at times. I remember thinking she would get us all into trouble – she seemed fearless. I admired her for that as much as it annoyed high-school me.

I was grateful to reconnect with her because I needed to be inspired by her fearlessness while I was facing my own fears about changing my life. Here was my chance to build an adult friendship with this woman I admired and regretted that I did not keep in my life.

When she told me about her battle with breast cancer, I was floored. I was angry. How can this happen to PAULA? Even though I wasn't a close friend, she was an amazing woman who inspired me. How would her family and friends get along without her?

Paula passed in May 2010. It's impossible for me to describe the impact the end of her life had on people I knew and her friends and family I never met. I hope you have known someone like Paula. Someone who was so full of life that they made you feel like you needed to live bigger, too.

During the few conversations we had over her last year, I was reminded of her courage. I felt it. When I looked at my current situation, I was ashamed that I let my fears and insecurities stop me from asking someone to teach me how to lift. How could I be afraid to do something so small when I had this example in front of me a woman who lived on her own terms? I had watched her do it since she was a teen. How could I possibly be such a coward about doing something so simple as hiring a trainer?

June 2010: Hired a Trainer and Started a Blog

"What are your goals?", Trainer Nico asked.

"I want to compete as a bodybuilder when I'm 50. I need you to teach me how to lift like a man." I replied.

"When will you be 50?" he asked.

"In two years", I said.

"We can do that. If you said, 'next year', no. But two years is doable.", he said.

I was old enough to be his mom, or he could have been one of my students - in fact, he was referred to me by one of my former students - so that's how I saw him at the time. I decided that to learn what I wanted to learn, I needed to be trained like a 30-year-old man. Never mind that I was a 48-year-old woman.

Felt guilty about spending money on myself again. But I knew I needed to pay for this because that was how I commited to things – don't waste the money! I promised myself I would not quit, I would not surrender, I would not let my inner "responsible adult" or other responsible adults around me talk me into making compromises that would derail me down the road. I had quit for the *last time*.

I would become a bodybuilder by age 50.

✳ That change in my mindset, goal, and training was the catalyst to begin progressing again with my health transformation.

Did It Work? Check My Data…

My 2008 lab work was done a year before I started my journey and the 2013 lab work was done a year after my first bodybuilding competition.

	2008	2013	Interpretation
Triglycerides	336	44	BIG improvement.
HDL (good cholesterol)	35	74	BIG improvement. Low risk for cardiovascular disease (CVD)
LDL (bad cholesterol)	115	154	Not a good thing, but my doctor said she wasn't alarmed since lab report about the size of the LDL particles was small.
C-Reactive Protein, Cardiac	1.6	0.2	Less than 1.0 indicates a low-risk for CVD
Insulin Resistance Score	Not checked	15	On a scale of 0-100 where 100 is highly insulin resistant. I'm highly insulin sensitive, which is good.

What Happened to Blood Pressure?

After a few dizzy spells over a month, I called and made an appointment to see my doctor about changing my blood pressure medication. The news was better than expected. With a big smile, my doctor looked at me and said, "no one ever comes off blood pressure meds". She was thrilled and proud! So was I. Took 17 months of proper self-care to get off those meds and that was my first goal. To this day, that's the one I'm proudest of reaching.

What Happened to Bone Mass?

From DXA scans done from 2011 until 2013, my bone mass increased by 1%. Considering I was going through menopause at the time, I should have lost between 3% and 5%, not gained. This is just another testimonial about why women my age need to lift weights.

I believed the change I needed to make was going to happen <u>one cell at time</u>. I think that's reassuring. It means that rejuvenation is possible. I had to be patient. I knew that, but still had some impatient days. That's when the support of people I put in my life helped. Change happened. And now I'm living with the happy consequences of those choices. That's my truth.

But Can You Do It?

Please talk to your doctor before starting a program, but it just makes sense that if you start taking care of yourself consistently, you will have positive results. You're going to have different strengths and different challenges than others, but yes, you can improve. If you neglect your health, there will be side-effects of that consistent behavior. So, if you practice self-care, there will be side effects of those consistent behaviors, too.

Chapter 1 Notes

Can Damage from Self-Neglect Be Reversed?

Chapter 2

Motivation vs. Determination

"Commit to the LORD whatever you do,
and he will establish your plans."
Proverbs 16:3

"Impossible is just a big word thrown around by small men
who find it easier to live in the world they've been given than to
explore the power they have to change it. Impossible is not a
fact. It's an opinion. Impossible is not a declaration. It's a dare.
Impossible is potential. Impossible is temporary.
Impossible is nothing."
Muhammad Ali

Changing your health is like planting a garden from seed. You prepare the soil. You plant seeds. You provide essentials like water, sunlight, plant food, fertilizer - the stuff those little seeds need to sprout. You tend the garden consistently while waiting to see something happen. It may take days or weeks before seedlings appear. And then you start new habits to protect them from the elements. Need to pull those weeds. Need to watch for bugs. But there are elements you can't control, like the weather, that will provide obstacles for the gardener. Eventually, there will be something to harvest, but that harvest doesn't happen in a week or two. It's nature and gardeners know what to expect.

Tending and waiting. Tending and waiting.

I don't see many people with the discipline to tend to their health like a garden. They get bored and switch programs thinking it's "not working". The truth is that it IS working, it has to work because it's our biology and scientific principles apply. But the changes are so small at first that we don't see them and don't believe in them. We need to change a LOT of cells before we see results in the mirror or on the scale.

I started with this core-belief:

My health problems are side-effects of my consistent behaviors.

Then I flipped that script:

Consistency works. The changes I want to see will also be side-effects of my consistent behaviors.

It takes nature time to change your whole body one cell at a time. Are you <u>determined</u> to change or just motivated? Motivation is fickle. Determination, discipline, consistency, grit, grind, habit…those words describe the mindset needed to practice self-care like a gardener.

It's hard at first – accept that and push through that part. Can't tell you how long that part will be – takes as long as it takes. The first <u>year</u> (not week, not month – *year*) was the worst for me. Sheer force of will got me through the first phase until the habits were so ingrained that NOT working out and NOT logging my food felt weird. Now, lifting is my coping mechanism. Food is still a bit of a challenge at times because I'm human – food provides comfort and is part of celebrations. But mostly it's fuel. Took some time to see things that way.

When I reflect, I think my program worked this time because I didn't count on feeling motivated. Can't lie – feeling motivated is fantastic! But it's a *feeling*. It's not going to be as consistent as you need to be if you're going to change your health. Adult responsibilities are real things. Obstacles will come up –

sometimes we create them, too. If you're trying to do something epic, life will fight back to maintain the status quo. Plan for it like the gardener plans for weeds and bugs.

What follows is how I planned to handle life when I was wasn't motivated. How would I tend my own garden? How would I prepare for the elements?

How I Turned Motivation into Habit

I changed my life 470 weeks ago at the time of this writing. For my entire adult life before that, I didn't stick with any kind of fitness or nutrition program. And I wasn't an athlete in high school, so it's more accurate to say that I stopped exercising regularly when recess and PE weren't scheduled parts of my day.

So how did I make this change? What did I do to make it work? I knew I needed to be organized to help myself stick to the plan until the habits were set.

First, I identified everything I could think of that would derail me on a daily or weekly basis. Then I made a plan to address each one of those things. I accepted that I had to have routines. I anticipated that I might need to tweak the plans. As a teacher, I'm a professional planner. My mindset was to use that experience. If I could facilitate and manage 30+ teenagers at a time, I could do this.

Obstacle 1: Work will interfere with workouts.

Couldn't get around the fact that the only time of day I could lift without distractions was during early mornings. That kept my evenings open to be at home with my husband and got the lift in before the teaching day started. For most of the nine years I've been training, my alarm went off at 3:30 am. I'm a teacher, so afternoons are unpredictable. Plus, I was an introverted teacher so my energy at the end of the day was always depleted. It didn't matter how much sleep I had – the activity of teaching and the noise of a high school wore me out.

I promised myself to work only during work hours as much as possible. That meant that I had to give up anything that took up my time that wasn't directly related to doing my job. That is a BIG decision for a teacher. That one impacts my colleagues and administration. I prioritized lesson planning, grading, and working with kids and started to say "no" to everything else. I didn't serve on committees. I didn't attend extra-curricular events - and that was a sacrifice because I know how important it is for kids to see their teachers at their games. I've graded papers on a stationary bike. And if it took me longer to get papers graded, it just had to be OK. That's just the way it's going to be.

Obstacle 2: No any healthy food ready to eat.

Food preparation was a critical new habit to establish. I knew that if I didn't do it, I would either skip meals or eat whatever I could find at a high school – which wouldn't be the fuel I needed to do what I was attempting – that "be a bodybuilder by age 50" thing.

I cooked breakfasts and lunches for the whole week during one afternoon on the weekend. I didn't vary the menu from day to day for most meals. I bought a microwave and compact refrigerator for my classroom. I also purchased a second food scale that I could keep at work. I would haul my food in "family style" and measure it out and heat it there. I kept preparation simple. Sure, it was boring. But I felt great, and I was healthy. That's more important to me.

Was I motivated to eat the same stuff all the time? No. But if that's all I had prepared, it was easy to log and easy to stay on track.

Obstacle 3: I'm too sleepy in the mornings.

A routine to deal with this obstacle was to pack my gym bag at night. If I tried to skip it, thinking I would do it in the morning, I usually forgot to pack it at all and ended up driving home after my workout to get dressed there for work. Some teaching days drained me so much, and I knew I didn't want to deal with this chore later, so I would head straight to the bedroom when I got home from work and packed it right away for the next morning. I've learned the hard way that it's smart to keep extra underwear and socks in that bag, too. I kept my shower towel in my car. I confess - I store a lot of extra stuff in the car. It's my rolling locker.

Obstacle 4: I don't have enough time.

Teaching demands a lot of time and we bring work home most evenings. Could I make my work routines more time-efficient? I was one of those teachers that spent hours researching and creating engaging lessons. I started there and reflected on that. Were my students learning more because they were playing with colorful, laminated cards I made myself? Probably not.

I gave myself permission to make lesson planning simpler and less time-consuming. For example, if I wanted my students to play a review game, instead of making an activity myself, I would ask them to write the questions and quiz each other. Turned out to be a <u>better</u> review activity. I learned that anything I could turn over to them almost always worked better than an activity I created. They were more engaged and less passive. What started as an effort to be more efficient with my time, ended up making me a better teacher!

Eventually, I reworked everything about my classroom instruction and procedures so that students were in charge of their learning. By the time I retired, my systems had run so smoothly that I left on time every day with all teaching tasks complete. I rarely brought work home.

I also found pockets of time by simplifying my makeup and hair routines. Over time, I just gave up on this stuff altogether. Less stuff to haul around and less time needed to get ready for work. People became accustomed to my new appearance without makeup and perfect hair.

I know what many women are thinking – "No way! I can't go out in public without makeup!" Yes. Yes, you can. But it's not about makeup and hair – it's about time. If time is the obstacle keeping you from working out, and you're reading this book to learn how I did it, then I'm going to tell you what I told myself - you <u>need</u> to find the time.

Prioritize how you spend your time and start cutting things out. What are those things you spend time on that you really don't need to do? If wearing makeup is part of your self-care routine, make it a high priority. But if your life is full, and you want to add something to it, something has to be dropped to open up the time.

When I first started, I chose lifting over makeup and hair routines. When I felt I needed to add Bible journaling as morning routine before going to the gym, I gave up a little sleep. And, when things got really busy, I started showering at night. I've had days when I wore black yoga pants when lifting so "getting ready" was just quickly changing my shirt for work. Might not work for your situation, but the point is to think creatively about where to save time.

Obstacle 5: I can't stick with it.

Every life-routine I've described here was developed to remove the reasons why I never stuck with a program. This time, it had to work. This time _had_ to be different. I promised myself that I wouldn't miss a day. Ever. In the first 140 weeks, life happened a few times, and I had had to miss a couple of workouts, but just a couple. When it happened, I didn't let myself make a judgment about it. Just got back to it. If you accept that this is your life now, you don't skip workouts – you reschedule them. Stick to the program. Keep moving forward. Progress continues even though some days need a "pause" button.

While I was working on this book, I reflected on the idea of "motivation" and realized it would be exhausting to feel motivated all the time. What keeps me going is the *process*. I love pushing myself. I love lifting! I enjoy looking for connections between training, nutrition, sleep, stress, and what my body does under certain conditions. It's all so miraculous to this former fat-chick who used to think that two plates of nachos with a couple of mixed drinks was a good dinner.

I love that the more I learn, the more questions I have. I love that every person's body is different and what works fabulously for one doesn't work we well for another. This is just really interesting! I know that weight training is something everyone should do for self-care, but most people aren't interested enough to train like a bodybuilder. Find the activity that brings you joy! I believe that for humans to feel good, we must move. The body is a "bio-miracle" that functions optimally when it gets to move regularly.

Chapter 2 Notes

Motivation vs. Determination

Chapter 3

A Life Remodel – How to Make it All Work

"Commit to the LORD whatever you do, and he will establish
your plans."
Proverbs 16:3

"Those who think they have not time for
bodily exercise will sooner or later have
to find time for illness."
Edward Stanley

My mother died when she was 56. At the time of this writing, I am also 56.

Mom died from a brain aneurysm. The doctors thought it might be congenital and asked if I wanted them to perform an autopsy to find out I might be at risk for one, too. Would you want to know if you had a time bomb in your head? I decided I didn't want to know. In hindsight, I don't think that was a good decision. I've lived my life since a little paranoid about it. If I get dizzy, I worry. If I get a headache, I worry. I've lived since then thinking that I might have limited time, too. No one knows, right?

The day I wake up that was one day longer than her life, I'll feel relieved.

Each day I do wake up is a blessing. Not in a "social-media-meme" way, but I feel truly blessed that I had that ER visit and was given a epic reality-check.

To start this chapter about a "life remodel", I'd like to invite you to start there. Your life is a blessing. It is a gift. It matters that you are here. I'll get to the nitty-gritty details about how to make all these new routines work, but the remodel MUST start with how you choose to live.

We aren't immortal. Our time here is limited.

Living like I'm on borrowed time has made me more grateful, less patient, less tolerant of people being rude or disrespectful, courageous, willing to set boundaries between "work" and "life", and more determined to practice self-care.

Is this a midlife crisis? Maybe. But it's been good for me, so I'm rolling with it.

How to Afford It

Let's deal with the pink elephant in the room right away – you will have to spend some money to do a health transformation. And for those of you who say you can't, I'm going to challenge you on that. If you're reading this book or following me on social media, and you haven't started yet, you know you want to do this. How you do it is up to you, but if you need help, figure out how to get it. Or figure out why you don't think it's important enough to make some hard decisions.

I used to feel guilty about the cost of a gym membership, paying for gas to drive to the gym, and that guilt it was an obstacle. How could I make that work? When I looked at our budget and saw how much I was paying for medication, doctor visit copays, and then that ER visit – all to treat something that I could fix – I realized that I was spending the money anyway. Our budget wasn't an obstacle – it was an excuse.

My husband and I made changes to our budget to make it work. If we were spending money on something that didn't support our goals, we nixed it. We ended up saving a lot more than the $60 per month we needed for two gym memberships and the gas required to drive to the gym. Netflix and YouTube replaced more expensive cable tv. We didn't eat all organic foods, just a few. We used thrift stores more than retail. We cut back on eating out and going to movies. When the lawn mower needed to be replaced, my husband bought a used push mower. Cardio!

When I started, working with a trainer was the most expensive part. There are more options now. If I were starting now, I would still consult with a trainer at first. Anyone starting in an unconditioned state needs a solid foundation. It's critical to learn how to lift with proper form, and the most efficient way to do that is to have someone right there helping you make adjustments. The next best thing is to work with someone online. Online coaching is usually more affordable than personal training. If you're willing to do some research, there are thousands of free demonstration videos online.

Think of it this way – you are willing to pay for some things to make your life better, so figure out how to pay for this, too. The follow-through? Yes, that's another thing. I'll refer you back to the chapter on motivation and determination.

How to Get to the Gym

Whether you decide to go to a gym or use a home gym, you need to make time for it. Personally, I prefer to go to a gym. It helps me focus on what I need to do if I'm in a different building away from my "to do" list. If I had to do it at home, I could make it work. Many people, even professional bodybuilders, make it work at home.

In the beginning, I used to get hung up on the "when is the best time to lift?" question. I received some solid coaching that I'll pass along to you. Ready?

The best time to work out is <u>when it works for you</u>. Period. Any research out there about the optimum time of day to do specific activities doesn't apply to your real life if you can't go during that "optimum" time. It is also logical to assume that we aren't all the same. Our energy levels rise and fall during the day based on many factors. That said, if the only time you can get it done is when your energy is low, then you're getting it done when your energy is low. If there is only one option – take it!

Many people will go early in the mornings because it works best for their family and work responsibilities. They choose to give up a little sleep to make this happen, even though they know sleep is important. Other people have more time at the end of the day. Some couples like to go together. Some don't. Some have more energy in the mornings, while others want to go after work to unwind. Some people can fit it in during their lunch breaks.

I'm an early morning person. Teaching all day wears me out, and I can't lift with the same intensity that I can in the morning. And I found that lifting before teaching made me a happy, more patient teacher.

At the time of this writing, I have memberships at two gyms. One is a world-class lifting gym and I'm lucky that it's in my city. Just walking in there motivates a lifter, because when you look around, you will see bodybuilders, powerlifters,

Olympic-lifters, strongman competitors, and people who are training for general health. That is the gym that adopted me when I lost my trainer. My picture is on the wall there. That's my home gym.

A few years ago, one of those key-access small commercial gyms opened about a mile from my house. It's convenient. The atmosphere is not as motivating, but that's ok. When finances are tight, I keep the membership at the gym that's closer to home, but I don't quit. The cost of that gym membership is a fixed expense that replaced monthly payments for medications. That's a fair trade-off for me.

How to Make Food Prep More Efficient

When I first started, I did what I saw others do on social media. I posted pictures of all my prepped meals in individual containers, too. And then one day I realized I could do things differently. Honestly, I was annoyed with having to wash all those little meal containers!

I set up a mini-kitchen in my classroom. I already had a microwave there. I bought a larger compact refrigerator that had a separate freezer, not the little freezer inside the fridge, but real freezer on top. I bought a second food scale to keep at work. And I brought in a couple of small plates and some silverware to avoid buying paper plates and plastic utensils.

Once that was set up, I was able to bring food to work on Mondays in larger containers. I bought egg whites, scrambled the entire carton, and brought it to work to keep in the refrigerator. I'd roast vegetables and bring those in a large container. When it was time to eat a meal at work, I'd weigh out my portions with the food scale, warm it in the microwave, and used real dishes just like at home. It was easier to wash the dishes at work than to keep buying paper plates and plastic forks.

Chicken prep became quite a system. On school holidays, when I had extra time, I bulk cooked chicken, cut it into smaller pieces, then froze it. One quart-size bag of cooked, frozen chicken would be about a week's worth of lunches for me at work. One afternoon of chicken prep would set me up for a couple of months. I'd grab a frozen bag on Monday mornings, put in the freezer in my refrigerator at work, and when I needed it, I measured it out and thawed it in the microwave. This process saved me so much time!

When life happened and threw off food preparation plans, I would buy bags of frozen chicken strips, frozen vegetables, or spend the extra money on those pre-cut vegetables. I never used frozen meals, though. They were too small. I needed larger portion sizes of protein. My preference was to keep my meals simple because I was tracking macronutrients as part of my bodybuilding contest prep diet. Established habits were not changed. My preference was, and is still, to keep it simple.

Meal Planning with a Family

I'm sharing a few solutions that moms I know have used with their families:

- Use your foods as the primary food and add sides/sauces

- Make separate foods.

- Teach them to cook for themselves

What works for your family depends on the unique set of variables you have to balance. The key takeaway is to be flexible. Don't take an "all or nothing" approach because that will create an obstacle that can derail your progress. If you feel like you can't stick to your goals because your family won't eat what you need to eat, that's an obstacle that can be navigated with a change of mindset.

How to Be Social and Stick to Your Plan

My advice here comes from years of doing this wrong. I was the martyr no one wanted around because I talked too much about my diet. Or I skipped functions and missed out. Eventually, people stopped inviting me altogether. I felt alienated and deprived. I understand how it feels to be committed, but I didn't do a good job balancing that in social situations.

(If I make this sound easy, please know that it is not. It's another skill to learn like all the skills involved with changing a lifestyle. It's a challenge, so it helped me to have a coach to provide accountability as well as lessons about how to balance my fitness goals with life.)

So, my advice is to go! Have fun! Participate. Stay focused on the thought that your people care more about the time they spend with you than with what you eat or how much of it you eat. But keep in mind that social eating is an important ritual for humans so you will need some tools to navigate this successfully:

- Unless you are competing in a bodybuilding show in a few weeks, don't pack your own food.

- At a restaurant, order something that most closely fits with your plan.

- Don't feel you need to explain why you ordered what you ordered other than to say it looked good, then change the subject.

- If you are at a function at someone's home, eat what they are eating, mind your portion sizes, skip some things, go for veggies, etc.

- Or choose to enjoy yourself! One meal isn't going to derail you. If you've been compliant with your program up to that day, and get back to it the next day, call it a refeed and relax. I'm serious – there is a benefit to your program to have a bit of a break. Your body will probably respond well to the extra calories. If you are worried about binging, then realize that is your challenge for the day, accept it, and meet it! Use smaller portion sizes. It's your choice whether to relax or use willpower. Beating up on yourself about your choice will be more damaging than anything you eat.

- Choose how you want to handle it, relax, and enjoy the time. Be loving toward yourself. This isn't going to be the thing that takes you off track. Trust yourself. Your habits will kick back in tomorrow.

- Keep this in mind – this is your choice. Unless you want to skip all social activities, you need a strategy that works for you and doesn't make your family and friends uncomfortable. Make it a win/win!

Logging food was the hardest new habit for me to establish. Unless you want to use a notebook, I would suggest using an online app. There are plenty to choose from, so if one isn't easy for you to use, look for another. Make sure the app you select tracks macronutrients – protein, carbohydrates, fats. I'm assuming most readers are interested in losing fat and increasing lean mass. Nutrition plays a vital role in this process and manipulating the macronutrients is how you, or your coach, will dial in a combination that works well for you and is sustainable.

When you pick your logging program, please understand it will take some time to learn how to use it. It will get easier. It will become a habit. But I won't lie – even with the help of a nutrition coach, the food preparation and logging habits took the longest for me to nail down. Measuring, weighing, and logging food can also be a bit stressful when you're used to not thinking about it. Again, it gets easier. And over time, you might be able to transition to eating intuitively because you'll follow the same patterns established when logging.

I've used online logging apps since 2009. I'm not an expert on all the apps available, but I've learned a few general hacks that have helped me stay consistent with logging.

- Create a list of "favorite foods". Picking from a short list is faster than searching the full database.

- Create recipes for common meals. For example, if you have a favorite lunch combination, create a recipe called "Lunch". When you log, you choose "Lunch" instead of each item separately.

- Standardize portion sizes. For example, I usually weigh out 80-85 grams of any meat for each of my three main meals. (Nutritionally, this amount will be about 25 protein grams.) Over time, this makes it easier to eyeball your portions if a scale is not handy. Also, if you can't log right away, using your normal portion sizes makes it easier to record later. Even if you're guessing, you know you always use at most 85 grams of meat.

- Use the "copy day" option if your tracker has it and your days are similar. Copy, then edit.

- Log the day ahead of time. It is faster to go in and edit at the end of a busy day. I used this hack on busy works days that had lots of meetings. I also found that it was easier for me to pass on unplanned snacking if I had already logged my food.

Patience & Priorities

Some weeks will go smoothly. Some will not and that's OK. When the negative self-talk starts – and it will - keep going. Your ego can rattle on and on about why you should quit while you go out there and do the things you promised yourself you would do. The "this will never work" loop can play on while you're doing food prep. Just do the food prep! These habits will win the day. I've managed to get on stage five times to compete as a bodybuilder even though my ego still tells me I have no business being up there as an "old fat chick".

Your program will not be done perfectly. There will be perfect days, sure, but perfect months? Probably not. We're busy adults. Self-care is a priority, but we have other priorities, too. Life happens and that's OK. It will still work. What you do consistently, over months and years, is more important than occasional, even epic, deviations.

The goal is to make this new lifestyle sustainable and as balanced as possible.

For Teachers (And Anyone Who Works Too Much)

After my ER visit in 2009, I went to my school administration and asked that a couple of things be taken off my plate so I could have time to fix my health. They were supportive and helpful.

That lasted <u>one</u> school year. One.

That's when I realized that I needed to set some boundaries. For the last eight years of my career as a public teacher, I had to continue to set those boundaries. There are certain professions where people are expected to do more than they are paid to do. This creates a lot of stress as they try to balance their commitment and passion with their health and families.

I published this blog on May 15, 2014. I want to include it here to finish this chapter on making it all work. Sometimes, you can't. Sometimes you have to choose to let some of the balls drop – and this blog is about my struggle making that choice.

Blog: The "P" Word (May 15, 2014)

Hi. My name is Tammy. I used to be a workaholic.

I'm not anymore and I suspect that annoys some people. Since I'm a teacher, I'm often expected to do things that have nothing to do with teaching and a lot to do with bureaucratic reports - lots and lots of paperwork. Or I'm expected to spend 50-70 hours a week getting everything done even though we are only paid for 35 hours. Sadly, most of what is expected distracts us from providing effective instruction. We are not provided the time or support we need to do what needs to be done. Spouses of teachers can attest to this.

When I say "no, I can't do that" or "no, I don't have time", I can have the "P" word thrown at me.

You're not... P R O F E S S I O N A L

Usually, it's an attempt to guilt me into being compliant. I used to hear it from a female colleague who didn't like how I dressed because my clothes didn't fit anymore.

Being "professional" used to be important to me. But after my health-scare, other words are more important to me now...

wife
ethical
moral
honest
trustworthy
balanced
joy
healthy
happy

Back in 2009, the decision to take care of myself was hard to make. I had a lot of guilt about how it was going to inconvenience my husband and impact my teaching. I knew I would have to quit being the "go to" person at work. But it turns out that **I'm a better wife and teacher because I'm taking care of myself**. Not just better because I'm going to live longer, but really BETTER. I'm more patient. I'm more creative. I'm more effective as an instructor because of those things. I won't let myself become burnt out. And I won't internalize the guilt trip about being "professional". I don't have time to waste.

Every day for the last year, I've parked my car at school next to a memorial for a colleague who was just a few years older than me. She was a wonderful woman, loved by many in our community, but died too soon. She had a stroke at work. She spoke with me a couple of times about changing her habits but always ended our conversations by telling me she was too busy to change. She put everyone else's needs ahead of her own health.

She had a large memorial service in our gym and now has a lovely stone memorial on our football field next to a faculty parking lot. Every morning when I arrive and every afternoon when I leave, I look at it. I'm reminded that this job can kill you. I wonder if the administration had to park next to that memorial every day, would they internalize what it means? I wonder if my colleagues who drive past it every day feel the same way I do?

I still need to remind myself that I can't care about what people think about how I live my life. I only have to LIVE it.

Chapter 3 Notes

A Life Remodel – How to Make it All Work

TAMMY WHITE

Chapter 4

How to Help Others Adjust

"Be always humble, gentle, and patient. Show your love by being tolerant with one another."
Ephesians 4:2

"Don't let the noise of other's opinions drown out your own inner voice."
Steve Jobs

When you begin a life transformation, people around you may become uncomfortable. Some will be supportive. Others will be critical. Others may be fearful. This may not be what you thought would happen. You expect support, you need support, but instead, you may find yourself having to help others come to terms with your decision to fix your health. It is important to know that you may have to help others understand what you are doing and why. It's important to know that you may have to commit to your program even if support from others isn't consistent.

I'm not saying people won't support you, but I am sharing what might happen over time as you're doing this work. It helps to get an idea of what "normal" might look like.

Your Marriage

Some spouses are fully supportive. Maybe they have already started their own health transformation and have been patiently waiting for you to be ready. Other spouses may worry about how your decision to change will impact the relationship. Will you expect them to do it with you? Will you spend less time with them? How will it change the routines at home? Will you drift away?

Your partner may need more reassurance from you that you're not changing your feelings for them, or your commitment to the marriage – you are fixing your health. You will be a happier, healthier version of yourself.

Your life together had patterns and routines. It's unsettling to one when the other starts to change. I didn't ask permission to make this change, but it needed to be discussed.

My husband was in the chair next to my bed in the ER. We were both scared. He knew why I needed to change.

Your spouse may need to be reassured that you don't expect them to do it with you. That's fair. This is a personal decision and you can only make it for yourself. Do not expect your spouse to change with you. Your spouse still gets to eat whatever they want to eat, and they get to keep it in the kitchen you share. This is <u>your</u> journey. If part of that journey is to learn how not to eat trigger foods your spouse still wants to have on hand, that's what you have to do.

Be empathetic and patient. They may never join you on this journey. Or they may see your progress and want to start.

The Unexpected Negative Comments

At first, there will be a lot of support from almost everyone. They want to be encouraging.

It will take a couple of months for people to notice a change in your appearance. And when they see your consistency is working, there will be compliments. As time passes and it becomes evident that you aren't going to give up, people might start making rude comments without intending to do so.

I don't know anyone who experienced a transformation who hasn't had something said to them that hurt their feelings. I'm not an expert about why people make negative comments. I suspect it comes from a place of insecurity. Maybe just having you there, standing in front of them getting it done, is just a reminder that they aren't getting it done?

When these comments start, it's hard to know how to process them. After a while, I learned to smile and change the subject. It's not personal. They are uncomfortable. Sure, I was annoyed. It was hard to handle when I got rude comments from someone close to me. But I reminded myself that they were uncomfortable.

The Food Pusher

"Really, ONE cookie won't hurt."

There is usually one person at work or in your family who is a food pusher. It's how they show affection. This is especially true for the person who bakes. Remind yourself that there is love in those cookies. Assume best intentions, not sabotage.

I've handled this situation several different ways with different levels of success...

I've handled it poorly. I gave lengthy explanations about my program and why I can't eat that cookie. (This is usually interpreted as being a judgment about cookie eaters and creates resentment.)

I've learned to handle it graciously. I thanked her for baking the cookies and expressed my appreciation for the hours of work it must have taken. Then I changed the subject to something engaging that's happening in the office, walked out, 'forgetting' to take a cookie.

When I could, I've handled it with balance. Ate the cookie, enjoyed it and adjusted my intake over the rest of the day if necessary.

Friends and Social Events

Full disclosure – I'm not a good role-model for how to handle this situation. To get everything done each day I wanted to get done, I was busy until I was too tired to do much more than go to bed. I also need a lot of quiet time to recharge because I'm an introvert, so I was never very social in the first place.

Because I've mishandled this, I can tell you what happened so that you can do it differently.

I've lost friends. They weren't close friends, but still relationships I regret losing. The time spent together was based on eating and drinking. When I stopped those things, we stopped hanging out. I'm sure they were relieved I wasn't there, because back before I prioritized balance, I was a food martyr. And a jerk about it at times, too.

To be fair, it seems like a lot of us go through this martyr-phase in the beginning. I needed to do it. The lifestyle change I was making was so big that I needed to recommit to it frequently. I hope that you can learn from my mistakes, be committed and passionate, but avoid the "be a jerk" part. I've since learned that to sustain my new lifestyle, I need to be more flexible in my food choices and in my relationships. It's up to me to be flexible because I chose this life.

The Back-Handed Compliments and Unsolicited Advice

"You look great, but you looked better when you were heavier."

"You look great, but you don't look professional." (Clothes didn't fit well anymore. Also stopped wearing makeup to save time in the locker room.)

"My friend did <insert a program or product>. *You should try that."* (Usually suggested because they didn't understand bodybuilding and thought I just wanted to lose weight.)

I got back-handed compliments when I first started my transformation and people could see my weight loss. I would just say "thank you" and leave it at that. The comments were awkward. Again, I assumed the best intentions. If they meant it to be an insult, that didn't matter. My progress was my own and opinions about it did not matter.

Now that I've been at this while, people have become accustomed to it, they understand what I'm doing, or it's obvious I'm not going to quit at this point.

As far as the free advice, try to avoid engaging in those conversations. If what they are suggesting sounds interesting, research it. But getting advice from too many people is like having too many cooks in the kitchen. It can be overwhelming.

The Doubters

"You're not going to be able to do it. Be realistic."

You'll have doubters. You're not imagining it. It may be family or friends. It may even be your trainer. I ran into it quite a bit in the first couple of years. These aren't haters – they love you. They are worried that you will be disappointed if you set a crazy, big goal and don't reach it.

What they don't understand at first is that the only way you won't reach your goal is if you quit. Sure, you've quit before. But you won't quit this time. Promise yourself. Promise your people who depend on you. Promise God.

No quitters allowed. Not this time.

I wanted to share this blog post with you here. I just competed in my second bodybuilding show when I wrote this one as an unsent letter to the trainer that dumped me eleven months before my first show. I'll tell you more about that in the chapter about setbacks. That was a big one.

Blog: Your Doubts Fueled Me *(June 26, 2013)*

> "There will be haters, doubters, non-believers and then there will be YOU, proving them wrong!" *Unknown*

Dear Doubters: I only think of you after I've accomplished something. I told you I would do this. I asked for your help. I told you I was serious and committed. But you did not believe me. You didn't believe <u>in</u> me.

I wonder if you have any idea what a colossal error in judgment that was? Do you realize that being jaded and short-sighted hurt me? But I used that pain as fuel when I had nothing in the tank. There were several mornings when I didn't want to get up at 3:30 am to head to the gym, but the thought that you might be right helped me swing my feet to the floor and get out the door.

While your doubt was an error from your perspective, and painful and confusing to me at the time, I'm grateful for it now. How things unfolded for me is well documented. I hope you learned something from your mistake, but I doubt it. Egos interfere with learning some lessons.

Creating a health transformation is hard. On the bad days, we feel like we need support from people in our lives. Family and friends may be able to offer that support, but there will be days when they aren't able to do that. Maybe some won't ever be able to support you. There may even be times when you will be their support if they are feeling anxious. We each have our own situations to handle but know that it's normal to have less than consistent support from family and friends.

Your journey is yours. Some people will understand what and why you are doing it. Some won't at first, but they will come around. I've lost a few acquaintances because what I was doing was too different than what I used to do. I changed. I own that. It's a fair and accurate claim to make. What is also true is that more times than not, I must be my own motivator out of necessity. Relying on people around you to be 100% on board with your goals 100% of the time is probably not going to work out well. Be patient with your people as they adapt to how you are changing. Be patient with yourself, too.

Chapter 4 Notes

How to Help Others Adjust

Chapter 5

How to Handle Setbacks

"I can do all this through him who
gives me strength."
Philippians 4:13

"You may not realize it when it happens, but a
kick in the teeth may be the best thing in
the world for you."
Walt Disney

I've had two kinds of setbacks – predictable and unpredictable. Continuing with the nature analogy, the predictable setbacks are like the thunderstorm that blows in during your picnic. They are predictable because they are universal. Everyone who has attempted to change their health has experienced some variation of these kinds of setbacks. That doesn't mean they are easy to deal with – they can knock you off track if you let them.

My unpredictable setbacks felt more like the experience of standing in your yard, looking at the ruble that <u>was</u> your house after an earthquake. Do you rebuild or walk away? These are the ones you'll remember.

<u>My</u> predictable setbacks had more to do with my lack of patience about waiting for results. Feeling disappointed at times is a normal part of the process. Predictable setbacks are not part of my past because I still wrestle with them occasionally. It's part of the process.   And I'm not an expert at handling them consistently with grace and maturity. What I <u>am</u> good at is *not quitting*. Some days, "not quitting" is the best you're going to do. (Confession – there are times when I quit. I just start again right away. That counts as "not quitting" in my book. And this IS my book.)

There is a separate chapter on how to deal with negative thought loops right after this one because these two topics, setbacks and negative thought loops, are linked together.

How to Handle Predictable Disappointments – The "Grind"

What are predictable disappointments? A plateau, a lousy workout, a less-than-supportive family member, a rude comment from a co-worker, a minor injury, etc. So many things can be listed here. I'll address some things in later chapters when I talk about negative thought loops and social media. But for now, I'd like to offer some tips on how to train yourself to grind through them.

A Big Scary Goal – Make one.

A "big goal" like "don't die early" is clear, but not concrete. Something you can measure like "lose 50 pounds in 6 months" is a typical goal, but it can set you up for repeated disappointments when the weight loss plateaus, which will happen because that's how it works. Scale weight drops do not happen linearly over time. It is better to make the Big Scary Goal something you will *do*, like "run a 5K" or "compete in a bodybuilding competition".

Your Big Scary Goal (BSG) needs to be something that excites you a tiny bit more than it scares you. Each day, remind yourself that your strength, endurance, scale weight, or appearance are ***side effects*** of the things you do daily to train for your BSG. Focus on that BSG when you don't feel like training or measuring food. Focus on the BSG when the scale stalls or when there are social pressures to over indulge.

I know your goal might be something like "lose 50 pounds in 6 months". But if you're like me, you may have set that goal before. Then when the motivation wears off and the grind starts, six months feel like a long time. I had a pattern of setting goals and quitting. And each failure reinforced my belief that I could not do it. When I stopped setting a goal tied to a result and instead made goals about behaviors, I followed through.

Have a "Bad Day Plan"

Life happens. Things will go wrong. Plateaus happen, and results will seem invisible. That's normal – you are changing your body one cell at a time. Changing your lifestyle isn't a temporary phase. There is no finish line. This is your new life so there will be rough patches. There will be days when you feel motivated. There will be a few more days when you don't.

Be ready for the bad days. Have a plan. Read through this list for ideas about what to include in your "Bad Day Plan":

- Repeat daily (sometimes more a few times a day): "DON'T STOP TODAY!"

- Remind yourself that YOU are in control, you are smart enough to do this, and you can solve any problem.

- Learn about what you are trying to do. Learn about the physiological processes of fat loss, muscle gain, and metabolism.

- Set daily goals that are behavior-based, not outcome based. "Don't skip workouts", "log all food and beverages", or "drink a gallon of water". You can achieve behavior goals. When you do, you continue your forward progression and results follow.

- Take progress pictures. Hard at first, but very motivating to look at on the "bad days".

- Make a Facebook album of your favorite motivational quotes so you can read through them when you need them.

- Put notes on the bathroom mirror with the quotes that inspire you.

- Workout. I know – the thing you don't want to do. But it's essential that you keep this promise to yourself, even on the bad days. Once you're there, it will feel good.

Routines & Preparedness Will Save You!

There will be bad days, but your daily routines will guarantee forward motion when you're not really "into it" that day. If early mornings are challenging for clear thought, set things up the night before so you can get up, brush teeth, grab gym bag, and head out the door. I leave myself notes on the coffee maker the night before so I won't forget anything the next morning.

- Keep the daily routine going, if you can, no matter what comes up.

- Have food prepared and packed up ahead of time.

- Pack the gym back the night before with work clothes. Keep extra underwear in that bag, too, just in case.

Support System – This is HUGE.

The enormity of the task can be overwhelming. There will be days when you feel insecure and think you're doing everything wrong – which is probably not true.

If possible, spend a little money to get the tools and help you need. Maybe you need an in-person trainer. Perhaps you can work with an online coach. Connect with people, in person or online, who are doing something similar. When you need it, ask a friend or two to hold you accountable and to encourage you when you need it.

Many people who want to make a big transformation, may not have a reliable support system at home. That's OK. You can find them online – Facebook and blogs are great resources. Start your own blog to document your process. It doesn't need to be the best blog out there – it's like a diary. Sharing it is not necessary, but some people find the public accountability to be helpful.

Relax

If you are feeling defeated and tired, it might not be just emotions - you might be just tired. This is a physical transformation and the body is under stress. Sleep is a major component for recovery. The body needs it to follow through on the processes of fat loss and muscle repair. Try to get 8 hours every night. (Although, honestly, I hardly ever did during the week. I just know I was supposed to.)

If you've been in a caloric deficit for a few months, you might need a diet break for a few days. I'm not talking about cheat meals or going nuts. A diet break means to bring your caloric intake up to maintenance, where calories in equal calories burned. A diet break gives the body a little extra fuel to recover from weeks of the physical stress of being in a calorie deficit. After a break, fat loss will start again, and you will be surprised at how fast it happens.

Please be patient, loving, and forgiving with yourself. Consistency is what works, not perfection. Time is relative. It takes as long as it takes.

The Big Unpredictable Setbacks

Every so often, life lands a sucker punch. These are the setbacks you didn't see coming. We all have them. And we can all compare and see that ours isn't as big as someone else's. But if you are in the middle of a health transformation, these rough patches can knock you off course. These are the events I described as earthquakes. Memorable. I'll share my top "hits" (pardon the pun) and what I learned about the process, about myself, or both.

I've had a few of these since I started my new life. In hindsight, one was a real catastrophe. One was only a bit difficult but felt like a catastrophe at the time. And the third was not a catastrophe at all, but it was kick in the gut that negatively impacted my mental game for a couple of years. As I describe these events, I'm not listing them in chronological order, but rather, in order of how they impacted my commitment from least to greatest.

In 2014, my husband was in a car accident. This was the event that I would call an actual catastrophe. Luckily, he only broke his kneecap, but it could have been much worse. He couldn't drive for a few months and his car was totaled. Insurance paid off his car but didn't leave enough for a new one. Because he works from home, we decided to change things around in our lives and make a go of it with one car. To make that plan work, I had to transfer to a school closer to home and use the less-equipped gym that was about a mile from our house. When he could drive again and needed the car, I would take the bus to work. I make that sound so simple and matter of fact, but it was a year of adjustments to routines for both of us.

All things considered, that should have derailed me. But instead, my gym and food habits held firm. They provided structure I needed when everything else was changing. That is my new normal – the workouts help me handle stress. My coach stepped up, adjusted the program for the new gym, and provided accountability. If I didn't have him in that role, it would have been tempting to quit.

The lesson? Work the problem. Think outside the box when life changes drastically and significantly. Go with the flow and adapt. Lean into your commitment and trust your routines.

Back in 2011, nine months out from my first competition, all my plans were blown apart and I found myself without a trainer or a coach. This was the difficult setback that felt like a catastrophe when I was living it. I've been fortunate to work with some great trainers and coaches. But the fitness field also attracts people who are more ego-driven than service-driven. I had hitched my wagon to one of those without realizing it.

I was panicked! There wasn't any other trainer in that gym who had the experience to work with a competitor. As a novice lifter and first-time competitor, I wasn't confident about carrying on by myself. I would be able to work out, but I didn't have the knowledge to do a contest prep.

The other trainers in that gym suggested that I needed to join the lifting gym a few miles away.

I'm not sure I can adequately describe how intimidating it was to walk into that lifting gym and ask for help. It was an early morning, still dark in the parking lot. My stomach was in knots. I focused on my Big Scary Goal as I walked through the door and then up to the front desk. Feeling defeated, I explained my situation. They welcomed me. They told me not to worry. They would help.

When I was on the verge of quitting because I could not see a path to get to my goal, didn't think I would find help, these people came to my rescue. Just walking into that lifting gym was intimidating, but it was the best decision ever!

I should have quit then, but I didn't. I still work out there. To get to the gym floor, you walk down a long hall filled with framed photos of bodybuilders, power lifters, strongman competitors, and other athletes. When I started lifting there, that hallway motivated me each morning. I wanted to work to earn a spot on that wall. I did it! Proud to report that it's still there.

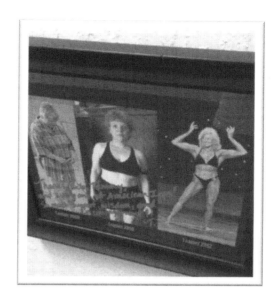

I wouldn't have made it to my first competition without the support I got from the people at that gym.

The lessons? First, trust your gut. I had some red flags about my trainer but chose to ignore them because I didn't want to start over. Second, ask for help and be ready to receive it, even if it doesn't seem like what you need at first. Trust that there is a plan and that the path you need to walk will become visible. That's faith. You'll need faith to get through a life-transformation.

Now the big one – the "nothing-burger" that became the most difficult setback for me to navigate because it hit me right in the tender spot where all my insecurities are stored.

At risk of sounding overly-dramatic, my 2015 competition experience <u>destroyed</u> my self-esteem as a bodybuilder. I almost walked away from a life I love because of this experience. That competition was the most humiliating experience of my life. Seriously – I can't recall any other event, even from the socially awkward years of high school, that compares.

However, it was also the catalyst for some of the most intense research about the importance of mindset in achieving hard things. This researched transformed my teaching practice. It transformed me more than the weights or the nutrition.

"So, what happened, Tammy?" you ask. Let me give you behind the scenes look at what it's like to step out on stage as a bodybuilder so you will have an idea about why this competition, on this day, became a setback instead of a celebration of my hard work.

The show I was at is a respected natural bodybuilding show in my area. It's a popular competition that draws competitors from around the world. I trained to be on that stage and was excited to be there. There were three classes for female bodybuilders that day – Masters (over 40 years old), Open (anyone who has competed before), and Novice (first-time competitors). I chose to compete in the Open class and not the Masters class. I could have done both, but it would be an additional cost. Turns out that most of the competitors in the Masters class also competed in the Open class, so I would have been on stage with the same women anyway- and the same woman won both classes.

For amateur bodybuilders, all the actual judging is done during the pre-judging round in the morning. Then we all come back for the night-show to do our individual routines and trophies are awarded based on the results from the pre-judging round.

During pre-judging, competitors line up on stage in numerical order based on our assigned competitor number.

Mandatory poses are called out by the head judge. The first four poses are symmetry poses where we face forward, right, back, left, and then face front again. After the four symmetry poses, they call out the other poses – front double-bicep, etc. At any point, the head judge may ask the competitors to switch positions in the line. The competitor moved to the center is likely in first place. Competitors asked to move to the ends are likely in last place and second-to-last place. If they are comparing two competitors, they will put them together at center stage so they can pose side-by-side. Competitors are compared to each other but also compared to a theoretical aesthetic standard for what a bodybuilder should look like.

All of this varies. I've seen first place finishers moved towards the end of a line just because the judges want to take a closer look at who will earn second and third place. When they move a competitor is telling, too. If they move you right away, it's likely that you've been put in last place right off the bat. If there are only a few competitors, they may not move anyone.

At this show, judges have been known to keep a line of competitors out there posing for as long as they feel it's necessary to assign placements. They also keep competitors out there out of respect for the sport – we worked hard to get there, and that stage time is the payoff.

We, as athletes, train to present the best version of our physique that day, but we also train to approach that theoretical aesthetic standard. That is why genetics plays an important part in this sport. Also, why posing is a skill to practice in bodybuilding – we pose to emphasize our strengths and minimize our weaknesses.

Imagine while one group of competitors is on stage, the backstage area is full of spray-tanned competitors hanging out, pumping up, or being lined up for their turn. (Fun fact – backstage is full of candy. We eat a little to help our muscles look full on stage. At this particular show, peanut-butter cups were the candy of choice. I wish I had gotten a picture of the wrappers in the trash. It was impressive!)

When it was time for the women's Open division to go out, we lined up just off stage in numerical order. I was the last of five women in the line for the Open class. Right behind me was the one and only Novice competitor, a 17-year-old.

It was fun to meet her considering she was the same age as my students. She was more excited than scared. A little nervous because she said she didn't think she did enough to get ready because she had to finish up her school year. My teacher-hat went on, and I reassured her that since she was the only woman in the Novice division, she wasn't competing with the five of us ahead of her in the line, but she was coming out with the Open class so she would not have to go through the pre-judging round by herself. It was going to be fun for her - no pressure. And it was fun for me because, as the oldest competitor in that line, a teacher, I would be standing next to the youngest, a high school student.

Our line walked out on stage, the lights were bright, and the house lights were low. I could only see the judges table and the first row. (Can't lie – going out there without my glasses helps with any stage fright issues. I can't see that far even if the lights are on!) Facing front, there were four women to my left, I was in the last position for the Open class, and the one Novice competitor, was to my right.

As we took our initial positions, we were introduced, and the audience was told that the first five of us were in the Open class followed by one competitor in the Novice class. It was explained to the audience that the two classes came out together so the Novice would not have to come out alone.

The head judge called out the four symmetry poses. We did each pose. We were asked to face forward.

I expected the next direction to be "front-double bicep", but it didn't come. We were holding our "front-relaxed" pose, which is anything but relaxed, and waiting.

The next direction was to ask me to switch places with the Novice moving her towards the center, putting me on the far-right end, *which separated me from the other competitors in my class!*

What just happened?

I was stunned for a second. I switched places as directed, tried to smile, reset my front-relaxed pose, but I was confused about why I was separated from the other competitors in the Open class.

If you assume they were following the standard practice for moving competitors, I was just moved a position that would be *less than* last place. It made no sense to me. At that point, I knew I just earned 5th out of 5 before we even started the mandatory poses, but I really didn't understand why I was asked to move at all. I was *already standing in the last place position* for the Open class when we lined up on stage initially.

We were out there for about 10 more minutes. Humiliated, I fought the urge to walk off. Instead, I claimed my corner of that stage and worked as hard as I could to get attention from any of the judges. The top three in the center were moved around a couple times. My hope was to be moved to the far-left side of the stage to stand next to the woman on the other end who was never asked to move. I assumed that meant she was probably in 4th place and I wanted a shot to pose next to her, so I could try to move up one place. I fought for that attention from the judges table, but I don't think anyone took a second look after I was moved.

When we were finished, I mustered some poise, walked off stage, headed straight through the backstage area, out an exterior door, and went straight to my bag that I left under a tree. I hoped to gather my stuff and get out of there quickly so I could decompress. And hide, honestly. I was so embarrassed! I'm not sure what just happened or why. At that moment, I wasn't confident that I would be a good sport about it because I felt humiliated. It happened in front of my husband, my coach, and an audience of athletes.

I threw sweats on over my posing suit, grabbed my bag and was ready to make my way to my car. When I looked up, someone was there to talk to me. Damn it! I knew this person, he's been involved in the sport for a long time, so I assumed he understood what just happened and wanted to make sure I was

OK. I know my memory of this conversation is not accurate because I was so emotionally flipped out when it happened.

"It's not your fault," he said. "You can't help your genetics. You can't change the width of your pelvis. Some people aren't built for bodybuilding."

What??? I did not see that coming!

Well, there it is. He wanted to make sure I knew that reason why I was practically asked to leave the stage was the width of my pelvis!? Good to know <insert sarcastic tone here>. I should have blown it off as an (insensitive) attempt to debrief my performance. But in that emotional state, my ego filed that away as the reason why I will always be put in last place, so why bother? I won't ever be competitive. I'm just a "wannabe" bodybuilder.

I respected this man, assumed he was telling me the truth, and didn't want to tell him that what he said was probably the most inappropriate thing to say to a female competitor who just walked off stage humiliated.

I don't remember exactly how I got out of that conversation – I suspect I was tight-lipped and said I needed to go. At some point over the next few hours, I would have to figure out how I was going to come back to the venue, get back on that stage to do my routine, and pick up my last place award gracefully. I did it. Honestly, I felt horrible, but there was no pressure at that point. It was just about doing the best I could do, smile, and then go eat pizza with friends.

Maybe I misunderstood everything? Perhaps the Novice competitor was changed to the Open class even though they introduced her that morning differently? When we lined back up that night off stage, she was excited and thought that maybe, because they had switched her with me, that she had earned a placing in the Open class. I thought that was a possibility, too. We were both wrong. She was awarded First Place, Novice class. I was awarded 5th Place, Open class.

If you're reading this thinking that I had lost all perspective about what's important, I agree. In my defense, competitions are physically and emotionally stressful. You train for them for years. You follow strict protocols that day about what to eat, when to eat it, when to add some salt, when to add some chocolate…all of it is science to make muscles look full and defined on stage. There are nerves. Hours of practice and yet, when you're on stage, you can forget any one of the dozen things you need to remember to pose the way you practiced. Then throw in the insecurities you fight back when you see other competitors. It's ill-advised to try to do anything that requires rational thought on the day of a show. And that's if it's going well.

I was in a hyper-emotional, fight-or-flight state the second they moved me to the right corner of that stage. Everything imprinted on my self-esteem like a branding iron. Every insecurity I had about being a former fat-chick who was too old to do this thing was confirmed. It was the nightmare of going to school in your pajamas – but on stage in a posing suit. Comments that were made to me with the best of intentions became the basis of a fixed mindset I still struggle against today.

The lesson? Despite how I let it affect me, the only thing that happened was that I was asked to stand in a different spot on stage. That's it. No catastrophe. The only thing injured was my ego. We can look at another person's experience and think "that's no big deal," but it is a big deal when your ego, left unchecked, fixes your mindset and the negative self-talk loop plays on repeat. "Don't try. Don't waste your time. You're a wannabe. You look ridiculous. You will fail and be embarrassed". These self-talk loops are a universal human experience. I'll get into this again in the chapter about negative self-talk.

This wasn't a real setback, not like the time my husband was in an accident or like the time I lost my trainer. I had done so much to get there. I literally fought to get my health back. I transformed my life. I've helped my husband believe he can do it, too. Strangers use my story as evidence that they can do what I did. These things are <u>so much more significant</u> than anything I'll ever accomplish in my sport.

But that experience, and those comments made to me about it, shook me hard. At the time, I wondered, "Is this the thing that will derail me?"

It damn near did. Every insecurity I've fought against since the day in 2010 when I walked into a gym and asked to work with a trainer was validated on stage that day.

Within a month, I was absorbing audio books about mindset, setbacks, and ego-management. My relationship with the sport of bodybuilding has become – complicated. Still working on that. I still don't feel like I'm part of that world. My competition experience reinforces my fixed mindset that I still haven't earned a spot and I don't belong there. To counter that, I've redefined what bodybuilding means to me. I'll still compete, but with no expectations. Training has evolved to be extremely personal and necessary for reasons that have nothing to do with placements.

I've competed twice since that show. When I did the same show in 2017, something funky happened on stage again, but I handled it better. My work in the gym improved my physique.

And my old-school inspired night show routine was a crowd favorite! This time, the unexpected feedback from another bodybuilder I respect was positive.

My current mindset is a bit more growth-orientated. Yes, I might always earn last place. I cannot control what judges do and another stage humiliation will always be a risk. I'm moving towards age 60 and I'm not sure how judges will deal with that. But I'll be up there in front of them for as long as I want to do this sport. I control what I do. I can be a better bodybuilder. I can improve.

My hope is that you might find something that sounds familiar when you read about my setbacks and the lessons I learned pushing through them. When you're in the middle of it, you might feel alone. You're not.

Four Steps to Handle Setbacks

The takeaway from this chapter is that setbacks, big or small, physical or emotional, are going to happen. Bears repeating – expect setbacks. They WILL happen. Plan ahead.

A strategy for dealing with them, no matter what they are, or how big they are, is the same...

1. Reflect and recommit to your success.

2. Adapt, don't quit.

3. Rely on your habits and routines.

4. Lean on your accountability system – that could be family, friends, online groups, trainer, or online coach.

Chapter 5 Notes

How to Handle Setbacks

TAMMY WHITE

Chapter 6

How to Handle Negative Thought Loops

"Trust in the LORD with all your heart
and lean not on your own understanding;
in all your ways submit to him,
and he will make your paths straight."
Proverbs 3: 5-6

"Fear is a habit, so is self-pity, defeat, anxiety, despair,
hopelessness and resignation. You can eliminate all of these
negative habits with two simple resolves: I can and I will."
Napoleon Hill

"I'm too old to do this. What the hell am I thinking?"

"My pelvis is too wide."

"I'm just a wannabe. I'm a joke."

"I'm too fat and won't get lean enough."

"I don't have enough muscle."

"I'm weak. Everyone can lift more than me."

"No one takes me seriously in bodybuilding."

Pause…breathe…focus…

You just read my most-played negative thought loops. This may be the hardest chapter for me to write and I've procrastinated it. By now, you know I'm not a writer – I'm a teacher who decided to be a bodybuilder. Most people think the scariest part of this decision was getting out on stage wearing a posing suit smaller than my underwear. That part isn't comfortable, but it's not too scary. The spray tan feels like a layer of oil, so I never felt too exposed.

What takes courage is acting in spite of your negative thought loops. To date, I haven't been able to shut them off, but I have learned how to mute them. And when I'm tired, worn down, hungry, or sad, I've learned to keep working even when I can't mute them.

Setbacks will happen. Obstacles will be there. They are real. The negative thought loops are generated afterwards by the ego. They are a defense mechanism. They are a psychological response to protect us from future harm of being embarrassed or looking stupid. If the ego gets its way, you won't do anything scary. It likes to stay safely snuggled up in a comfort zone.

My negative thought loops started I first stepped up and said, "I'm going to be a bodybuilder by age 50". But up until a certain point, I knew they were in my head and not reality. That changed in 2015.

After the 2015 competition experience described in the last chapter, that time when I was switched on stage with the 17-year old novice - the negative thought loops went into overdrive. A new one was added... "See? I told you it was true. You don't belong up there. You are a wannabe."

Sure, the experience happened. But I created a habit of reliving it daily. Every time I went to the gym to lift, I had a "why bother?" message running in the background. The next two years were spent reading and reflecting on strategies I could use to keep my mental game positive so I could continue my training.

I think I listened to dozens of audiobooks. Each book led me to the next. I learned about Eastern philosophy. I learned about historical figures who overcame impossible obstacles. I learned about how elite athletes are coached. I even learned about neuroplasticity – how our brains can create new pathways to adapt to trauma or to develop new habits of mind...like negative thought loops.

The most impactful books were the ones that addressed mindset and ego.

- <u>Mindset</u> by Carol Dweck

- <u>Ego is the Enemy</u> and <u>The Obstacle is the Way</u>, both by Ryan Holiday.

Most of what I learned improved my teaching practice. I finally understood what my struggling math students felt like in class when they just couldn't do it. They had a fixed mindset of "I can't learn math". I redesigned my classes so kids could learn at their own pace and have a clear expectation that they must keep trying after a failure. They needed experiences that would spark a growth mindset. Wish I could say I was able to reach every kid, but I couldn't. Fixed mindsets are impossible to break from the outside. The person must be willing to crack the glass from the inside first.

My fixed mindset about what I'm capable of achieving as a bodybuilder is reinforced by my negative thought loops. I know it. I'm still working on it.

My question to you – what are your negative thought loops? What fixed mindset are they supporting? Are you comfortably snuggled up inside your comfort zone? Can you find a way to crack the glass from the inside?

It takes a lot of courage to continue after a setback, not just because of the setback, but because it can fix your mindset that continuing is futile. That's when most people quit. That's when you will need to stand firm, find courage, and push ahead.

What I've learned is that the loops are predictable. They will start when I'm stressed. They will start when I'm tired. They love to get cranked up when I go to bed. (Love it. Negative thought loops are jerks.) I can mute them with movement – lifting always works. Walking while listening to an inspirational audiobook works, too. (I think I've listened to both of those Ryan Holiday audiobooks at least six times.) I have a playlist of motivational videos on YouTube, too. When I can't quiet the negative loops down on my own, I will ask a friend for a pep talk.

It is essential to have a clear understanding of your "why" for doing the hard thing you are working on. You need that core belief in place. When it gets hard – and it will – you need that touchstone.

What is your "why"? Why do you want to do this big thing that scares you?

My primary "why" is self-care. The discipline of training with nutrition to support my training renews me. I believe it saved my life. But I need a goal, so I compete as bodybuilder to give my training a purpose. It's not necessary to compete to practice self-care, but I love being a bodybuilder and want to go through the entire cycle of improvement, contest prep, and stage.

There is something else, too. It's humbling to think about how what I've done to save my own life has created a ripple effect. People I love believe they can change because I changed. Beyond my inner-circle, I never expected people in the world to pay attention. But they are. You are reading a book I never knew I'd write. My bigger "why" is how my story helps others believe they can do it, too.

When my negative thought loops get a bit too loud and I want to quit, I check in with my bigger "why". Someday I may retire from the sport, but I won't quit just because I started to believe my negative-thought loops.

What's your bigger "why?" Take a moment and reflect on it. You'll need it. It's a powerful antidote to your own negative thought loops.

To help you understand my "why" and my struggle with my negative thought loops over the years, here are the blogs I wrote as I worked through this difficult issue.

Blog: "Put Your Ego in a Box" (January 17, 2013)

There is that person who just won't...shut...up. Ever. They don't listen. They only wait for the next gap in the conversation to continue to "enlighten" the rest of us because we are clueless. Ignorant arrogance dripping all over the floor.

Do you know anyone who believes they know more than they really do? I was reflecting on this on my drive home from work today. I just want to tell them..."**Put your ego in a box, seal it, push it aside, and LISTEN. You have a lot to learn.**"

I don't know where "ego in a box" came from, but I like it. It just popped into my head.

Then I reflected. I made a mental list of the times when my ego was in my way. That led to the thought...

"Get out of your own way."

How often does THAT happen? For me? A LOT. I AM IN MY OWN WAY A LOT.

Concerning my own health, it wasn't the obstacles that stopped me - *it was what I thought about the obstacles.* I was the one in my way. Seriously, there were *good* reasons I didn't take care of myself. I could list them for you if asked...

- I have too much work to do.

- I can't afford the gas to drive to the gym.
- I don't have time.
- I don't like how that food tastes.
- I don't have clothes to wear to the gym.
- I don't want to look stupid at the gym.
- I don't want to work with a trainer because it will be embarrassing when they find out how pathetic I am.
- My back hurts.
- I don't have time to log food.
- I can't afford to buy the gadget I need.
- I need training, but I can't afford the training.

When I was finally sick and tired of being sick and tired, I decided to solve the problem instead of explaining why I couldn't solve the problem. So, I guess **I put my ego in a box**. I gave up and admitted I needed help. I tackled each thing. The "gas to go to the gym" was a big deal for me. I decided that it was just part of the necessary expense to get healthy. I rationalized that if I could get off my meds, that would help pay for the gas.

Ok, so that's it. "Put Your Ego in a Box" is my new catchphrase. I hereby copyright it. Hahahaha!

Blog: "Fear Revisited" (October 19, 2013)

My life is a constant struggle with fear. I'm sometimes wrestling with my own fear, or I'm trying to help other people wrestle with theirs. I've written about fear before. It's such a common experience many of us share, I wanted to write about it again tonight. Here is what I've learned about fear.

FEAR is a THIEF. How many people don't live the life they are supposed to live because they are afraid? Fear took my dream and left in its place a life full of safe routines. I used to cling to those routines like a security blanket. I "didn't have time" to go to a gym and risk looking foolish - the old, fat woman who moved awkwardly and couldn't do much very well. Fear ruled my life for too many years. My health suffered. I was not being who I was supposed to be.

FEAR is a BARRIER. It will stop you. It will change your path. I realized this after my mother died. After I started to come out of the fog of grief, I looked back at my life and saw a series of decisions made to avoid something. It was then that I made a promise to myself to not let fear define my life. However, I forgot about that promise as the years went by. Initially, my health transformation was about avoiding an early death - another decision based on fear. But then I remembered. I remembered my promise to myself. I remembered that thing that fascinated me when I was much younger, but I was too afraid of it to try ... bodybuilding. Once I decided to do it, I didn't see the barrier anymore. I just assumed it was going to be a lot of work.

FEAR is a CHARMING LIAR. "I can't afford it." That's what I told myself about getting the help I knew I needed. Heck, I told myself that about just driving to the gym. "I can do it myself." That's what fear told me. I was afraid to invest in myself. I was afraid to take the risk. I knew that if I faced my fear and took the risk, I would NOT let myself fail. I would NOT quit because that would make the money and time I spent wasted. Fear kept lying to me. "You can't do it. You're too old. You're too out of shape." I knew there was one thing I had to do to succeed - DON'T QUIT. It was going to work. I just needed to be patient and consistent.

Fear continues to whisper in my ear. I regularly have to push forward despite those little whispers. The strongwoman training and competition was a great example of how I battled with fear almost every day for 8 weeks. It wasn't whispering to me then - it was very convincing, very logical. I wanted to quit every day. I used a trick I've used before - I left myself notes on my bathroom mirror.

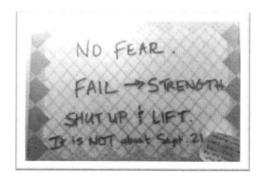

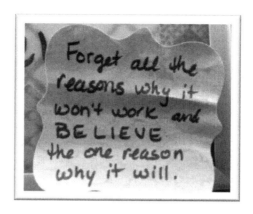

The first year of my journey was a struggle. I had to make myself get up every day and do the thing I knew I needed to do. It took a whole year before I fell in love with exercise. That's when I made the decision to do the thing that scared me the most - hire a trainer and learn to lift so I could become a bodybuilder. The exhilaration of being that bold and pushing through my fear propelled me. Everything I've accomplished since then is a milestone of another fear conquered. Doing a posing routine on stage? Yeah, that was a big fear.

I work with people of all ages now as they face things that scare them a little - or a lot. I'm either their math teacher, their trainer, or their coach. I try to offer a little courage when they need it. Some take it, some don't. They aren't ready. When they are ready, I'll be there. I ask them to acknowledge the fear and act anyway. Pretending it's not there is like pretending there isn't an elephant in the room.

I'm still afraid. However, I've learned that the most rewarding things I've done have happened when I act in spite of my fear. I love this!

BLOG: "The Importance of Mindset to Do Scary Things"
(June 24, 2016)

Still working on developing a consistently positive, growth mindset about when I compete again next summer. Now that it's a little less than a year out, nerves switched on this week. The self-discovery path I was set on because of that 2015 competition experience has changed my teaching practice and my life, I guess. For that, I'm grateful. Still, my "fight or flight" response gets a bit stuck in "flight" when I think about another sticky spray tan, posing suit, and stage experience. I told my coach this week that I've developed a little learned-helplessness about what I'm going to be able to accomplish in this sport. I call it that because I recognize in myself what I see in my students when they come into my classroom to take a geometry exam. "I'm going to fail", they tell me. What do I tell myself? "I've been placed dead last three times." "My pelvis is too wide." "My shoulders are too narrow." "I'm too old." All of these are my version of "I'm going to fail, so why bother? Who am I kidding?" And nothing anyone says is going to change 'reality', right? You know how this goes.

It's uncomfortable to admit, but we all do it at some time about something. That is a sign of a fixed mindset about one's ability to do a particular thing. Working towards a growth mindset allows for the "I'm not ready, but I can improve" attitude. Once I recognize it, I can deal with it. The trick is to catch it before I end up ruminating on it. I've been going back and forth on this one for almost a year now.

Thank you, readers, for hanging with me while I work through these things. I don't expect this to be resolved until after I'm on stage again. Oh and, I kid you not - as I type this, I'm watching a baby bird through the blinds of my window. She will be ready to fly soon and is tentatively exploring the opening and perch of her birdhouse. And... she goes back in. Not ready yet. Hope she doesn't decide there is no point...

Way back in 2010 when I first set my mind on bodybuilding as the "big, scary goal", I wasn't a person who had any business making a goal like that. Almost EVERYTHING had to be changed - how I ate, had to make time to train, and I had to retool all my routines about teaching because I no longer had time to bring work home.

I'm still married to the same wonderful man, but he was forced to make some adjustments because his wife just up and decided that she was going to be a bodybuilder now. What was I thinking? How would I do this thing?

The mental game was so hard then! Looking at what I've done, it seems silly to still be fighting dragons, but I've apparently developed a habit over the years of falling back into negative self-talk when I'm insecure and doubtful. Back then, I put a small bulletin board up in my bathroom and filled it with motivational quotes that meant something to me. Basically, I left myself reminders where I would see them to counter negative thoughts with positive ones. I think I will do that again. And I just happen to have a <u>bigger</u> bulletin board!

Something else occurred to me this morning while I was at the gym. It would be useful for me to mentally redefine what is real for me about being on stage and then rehearse those thoughts. I've competed three times. I know how warm it is under the lights. I know what it smells like - a mixture of spray tan and hairspray. I know what the stage feels like under my feet. I know I can't see much past the first two rows in the audience without my glasses (which is a blessing). I can completely visualize it now, which is a plus. My thoughts up there are loud. I can create a new set of thoughts to put with that visualization. When I got home from the gym, I wrote this out. I don't think this is final form. At some point, I'll print it, laminate it, and put it up on that bathroom bulletin board.

I'm here to celebrate.

I celebrate the joy and gratitude that I finally get to do this.

I celebrate the useful, purposeful pain that forced growth and renewal.

I celebrate the courage I found minutes ago to walk
out and stand here.

I celebrate the discipline to push myself to do things I could not do when I was a younger person.

What you see is the **PHYSICAL MANIFESTATION** of my **MINDSET**.

I've overcome obstacles to be here.

I've slain dragons. I got back up when dragons slew me.

See those people there? The judges? They have a task to do for the promoter of this show. I am not here for them and what they do is not my concern. I'm here, on this stage, on this day, for my own reasons.

I'm here for the people who love me, who inspired me, who helped me, who believe in me, and who need me to be here.

I'm here for my mom.

I'm here for the pictures that will document the inner strength the struggle built.

I'm here to show others how to slay dragons, too.

I'm here to celebrate.

Chapter 6 Notes

How to Handle Negative Thought Loops

TAMMY WHITE

Chapter 7

Social Media

"We do not dare to classify or compare ourselves
with some who commend themselves. When they measure
themselves by themselves and compare themselves with
themselves, they are not wise."
2 Corinthians 10:12

"Comparison is the thief of joy."
Theodore Roosevelt

Social media can be a useful tool for the person working on transforming their health. But it can also be a distraction and a source of triggers for negative self-talk. I hope by sharing my experience with social media, you can decide how to use it in a way that is helpful and be able to set healthy boundaries about how you use it.

What to Expect if You Want to Share Your Journey Online

The day I decided to set the "Big Scary Goal" of competing as a bodybuilder by age 50, I started the blog. The plan was that it would serve two purposes. It would be a journal to document my progress and struggles. And I needed the extra layer of accountability. It helped me stay on track because I made a public announcement that I was going to do this thing. Well, "public" is an exaggeration. If no one reads a blog, it's basically a diary.

To make my goal "public", I shared links to my posts as status updates on Facebook. That was a bit scary the first time I did it. If I didn't follow through, I risked failing publicly, too! That's the accountability at work.

After a couple months, I noticed that a few Facebook friends seemed to be appropriately annoyed by my overly enthusiastic fitness posts. (I was annoying. I own that. New converts to fitness can be too enthusiastic. Everything is "OMG!!!!! I feel soooo good! You should do this and stop eating those nachos!!!" I went through that phase. I'm over it. The world may now enjoy their nachos without my judgement. I might have some, too.) I created the Lifting My Spirits Facebook page so I could have a place to share my blog posts that was separate from my personal feed.

My first 100 followers were mostly my friends. I felt the pressure to "build the page" just because others were doing that. It was a bit like a game. But I didn't really have a plan to do much more with it other than use it to share blog posts and other things fitness-related. For a year, that's all that was going on – my friends and I posted on my little page. It was working for me because I'm an introvert and will get overwhelmed when there is a lot interaction. I keep my circle of friends small.

And then something wonderful and horrifying happened to this introvert in December 2013. I did it to myself.

I could lie and say I don't know why I did it. But I do. I saw a transformation picture on a much larger Facebook page about female bodybuilding and thought to myself "THAT'S a transformation? Well, this will blow your mind" and I sent off this picture…

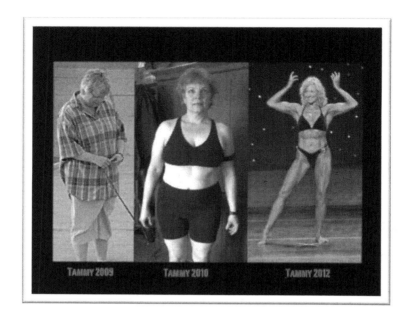

It was impulsive and ego-driven. Not my usual modus operandi. Up to that point, I had been cautious about keeping that image to myself. I had been asked to share my story on other pages, but I was apprehensive about doing it. I did not want a lot of attention. It was a dramatic transformation image, so some page administrators were more motivated to post it as "click-bait" and wouldn't monitor comments.

So why did I send it to that larger page on that day? I had followed the page for a while and knew the administrator was respectful to female athletes. He was protective. But what made me send it impulsively? Ego. I was feeling a bit feisty and full of myself. (It happens.)

I wanted to pull it back as soon as it was sent. And I spent a good 5 or 6 hours with a knotted stomach when I realized that the page administrator thought it might be a fake picture. Understandable, I guess. It never occurred to me at the time that people faked these kinds of pictures because I was a fitness social media newbie.

Once he did post it, my page grew like crazy. That photo went viral. I lost track of it. The reach was over a million people. It still pops up on Google searches. Saw it used once to promote a weight training class in Spain! (*As of this writing, I've never promoted products. If you've seen my image used to sell things, it was done without my permission.*) I'm on several Pinterest boards. I think that picture might still be floating around the Internet.

I've done interviews in blogs, in podcasts, and magazines. I was even interviewed by a local television station because the anchor's trainer showed her the picture and they didn't believe it was real, either. After researching it, they found out we lived in the same city.

I might be the only high school math teacher ever to have a full-page photo in a school yearbook – in a posing suit! Makes me smile now to remember the first time a kid asked me to sign that yearbook!

You may have first found my story through social media. That is a blessing to me. A HUGE blessing! Perhaps it wasn't *all* about ego when I sent that picture to that page. It's humbling to think that the ripple effect caused by that one impulsive act, something so out of character for me to do, has brought you and I together at this moment.

So, all that said, if you're thinking that having a large following on social media is a goal, we should talk about the negatives.

I miss being a private person. People forget I'm a real person and will drop all kinds of negativity into a thread of a post. Or, people assume that it is part of the game, I'm a target, and I must learn to deal with whatever rude comments they feel entitled to make – and that is 100% true. Anyone thinking about building a social media presence will need to develop the skill of being a bit disconnected from the negativity. That takes time, and sadly, experience. I honestly don't think anyone has thick enough skin to handle the hate that can come at you on social media. Some cope by not reading the comments. But I do read them. Every single one.

Early on, I decided that my social media presence would be one of positivity, humor, faith, and motivation. I needed to live up to the name "Lifting My Spirits". I manage my social media accounts like my classroom – expectations are made clear, people who are trolling are given a chance to play nice but will be banned and blocked if necessary. Because I've done that for years, my Lifting My Spirits social media accounts are not safe places for trolls. But it has become more work than I anticipated. The key takeaway for you – this is more work than it appears.

Occasionally, a follower will step over the line of simple trolling. They are bullies. My photos have been shared on other

Facebook pages and people argued about whether it was a fake photo. Some didn't care if it was real – they thought my "after" looked gross, disgusting, and it was important to them that they told me so. My image is an object and I've been treated as such at times. I've been cyber-stalked across different platforms. Clearly, something about my story triggered something ugly inside some people. I've been challenged and maligned. I've received some offensive messages with inappropriate requests, sometimes with photos. None of it matters. None of it changes the reality of my daily life.

The negativity I've described here is par for the course for social media fitness personalities. I don't even have a large following compared to others, so I'm sure their exposure to this dark side is exponentially greater than mine. I didn't know this would happen and was shocked by it when it started.

All in all, the positives greatly outweigh the negatives. Whenever I'm feeling a bit too vulnerable and think about pulling it all down, I hear from someone who says something I posted helped them find courage to make a change they needed to make. How can I tell you how humbled I am by that? I didn't know that was going to happen when I started my blog in 2010! I didn't think I was doing something other than fixing myself. This social media thing has grown beyond me now. It started as a tool to hold myself accountable - and it did precisely that. I've lost count of the number of times I've wanted to quit but didn't because I knew that telling my followers that I quit was going to be harder than figuring out a way to make it work.

Following Others on Social Media

Most people won't be social media fitness personalities. Most people don't want to be, either.

I'm going to be upfront here – I'm not an expert on which fitness personalities to follow online. I don't follow many. I follow my friends. Some of those people are in the industry, so perhaps that counts as following a "fitness personality"?

When I first started my personal transformation process, I followed more people online. People who had a lot of followers. I thought that meant they knew what they were doing. I was always researching. While looking for information about something, I'd come across someone who put out good content, so I would follow them. Most were coaches.

After a while, I noticed that I felt anxious and overwhelmed. I started second-guessing everything I was doing, even when working with my coach. I realized that I was being exposed to too much information.

If you follow too many people, you may start to lose confidence in your own process. If you catch yourself second-guessing your program when there isn't a legitimate concern, cut back on the information input. Success requires focus. If you're changing your program frequently, you won't have the results you want. If the input from the gurus online is making you feel like you're "doing it wrong", shut off the gurus.

If you can, hire a coach, focus on the plan, and grind. If you can't hire a coach, research and write your own program, but stick to it for months, give it time to work, and focus on progression within that program.

The most insidious effect of following people on social media comes from our natural compulsion to compare our progress, or our physiques, to those who post pictures online. If that makes you feel motivated – that's great! But pay attention to what you're feeling and what you are thinking. If images on social media trigger negative self-talk, it's time to decide if you really need those images in your life. It does not matter how anyone else reacts to it – we've all had different experiences and don't respond to things the same way.

It helped me to disengage. I deactivated Instagram for a long time. I stopped following almost all fitness pages on Facebook and started following more pages about other interests. More pages with crafts and jokes – fewer pages with selfies. I'm on a mission to ban underwear selfies in my feed. I'll let one or two go, but if there's no content and it's all about selfies, I'm out. If I'm not learning something, laughing, or feeling spiritually enriched, it doesn't need to be in my feed.

No one else is walking your path. It's going to sound cliché, but it's true – you're only competing with yourself. You control what you do, nothing else. If an image of another person's physique makes you think of what's possible and motivates you to stay consistent with your self-care, that's ideal and will help you reach your goals. If something about that image makes you feel like there is no point in trying – that's working against you and doesn't need to be in your life.

Usually, we see photos online that are a tiny-bit fiction. It doesn't make sense to compare our progress to those photos. My competition pictures aren't fake, but they aren't how I look in real-life, either.

Pictures of bodybuilders on stage are usually not edited, but they are also not pictures of a sustainable physique. To attain competition conditioning, we take fat-loss to an extreme that is not healthy to maintain for more than a short amount of time. Not only that, we do other things to create an optimal stage presentation. We manipulate carbs and water to make muscles look fuller and their definition sharper. We practice posing to emphasize our strengths. We also get a fake tan specifically formulated for competitors to keep us from looking washed out under the lights. That abnormally dark tan will also make us look more defined.

Many social media fitness personalities will use the same techniques to appear leaner for photoshoots. Some just take a ton of selfies when in that condition and recycle them for later use. Or they stand in some weird pose never seen in the real world to make their butt look better. Can you imagine how funny it would be if everyone stood around like that waiting to pay for groceries? Hilarious!!

One way to decide if following others on social media has been helpful or hurtful is to answer two questions:

1) Are your negative self-talk loops started when you scroll through social media?
2) Do you spend time practicing how to stand uncomfortably to get a good butt selfie?

If you answered "yes" to either of these, consider cutting back a bit. And that includes following me if what I'm posting is triggering something unhealthy for you. I hardly ever post selfies because 1) I don't want to, and 2) I don't think people need that from me. A sustainable physical transformation is only possible when done along with a mindset transformation, so I'd rather post something that is going to support positive self-talk and a growth mindset.

Think of your social media activity as a component of self-care. It's important to be aware of what is helping you and what may be causing you to lose focus. As you look at what others are posting, pause and reflect on how you feel.

When looking at an image, what are you feeling?

Positive Feelings	Negative Feelings
Motivated to be a better version of you.	Self-judgment
	Triggers negative self-talk.
Learn something from the content you can use.	Makes you critical of your lack of progress.
Made you laugh.	
	Bad energy. You feel insecure, annoyed, or angry.
Good energy. You feel happy.	

As in most things, how you participate on social media will change depending on the situation. There are times when you are busy, working under a little more stress than usual, so pulling back from social media will help you focus on what you need to get done. Later, you may choose to become more engaged.

Chapter 7 Notes

Social Media

Chapter 8

Eating 101

"But food does not bring us near to God;
we are no worse if we do not eat,
and no better if we do."
1 Corinthians 8:8

"I've learned that I still have a lot to learn."
Maya Angelo

I am not a registered dietician and make no claims to the contrary. Please consult with your physician before making any changes to your nutritional habits. Everyone's dietary needs and restrictions are unique. Readers are advised to take full responsibility for all their decisions pertaining to their health.

Want to stir things up on social media? Tell people how to eat. There are people with some strong opinions on this subject, just like politics. Some will give themselves permission to tell you how to eat and how to vote with equal passion.

But in the real world, people struggle with sorting through all the information. Companies pushing a program or a supplement take advantage of the confusion to promote their products as the "easy and simple" way to reach your goals.

Here's something you won't hear often, but it's needs to be said more. And it needs to be accepted and practiced...

You're not supposed to be on a diet all the time.
Fat-loss phases are a tool that should be used rarely.

That said, I know many people reading my book are looking for information about how I lost my weight. There is no "plan" to share. I learned how to use nutrition differently to reach my short-term and long-term goals. What I do now is sustainable and is part of my self-care physically. And that included creating a healthy emotional relationship with food.

I think my experience with dieting was similar to many others until I started working with a nutrition coach. I've done several of the named programs – Weight Watchers, Atkins, Rotation. I tried keto. None of these were sustainable for me. They were too restrictive with calories, food choices, or not practical for my real-life long term. But in 2009, my goal changed. I wasn't interested in just weight loss – I wanted to learn how to care for myself nutritionally. My mindset was that this wasn't a quick-fix, but the final fix. I was more focused on health. I wanted to <u>learn</u> about nutrition, so I could adapt when life threw curve-balls.

The reason any program will "work" if weight loss is the only goal, is due to biology – eat fewer calories than you burn, and the body will burn tissue to sustain life. Notice I did not say "burn fat". Yes, it will burn fat. But it can use other tissue, too. Our biology is designed to sustain life. If the caloric deficit is too high for too long, the body will also use other tissues as a fuel source.

When people say they want to "lose weight", most people are interested in fat-loss and want to keep as much of muscle, bone, and other tissues as possible. If you look at pictures of people who have been malnourished over an extended time, you can see that they lost a lot of muscle mass. What we can't see is that they have also lost density in connective tissues, organ tissues, and bone mass.

In the beginning, people are in a hurry. Anyone who has managed to sustain their transformation will tell you to win this game you need patience and balance. An extreme approach will not work over time. The weight will come back. If you don't care about that, if you're trying to lose 20 pounds by a certain date, are you willing to trade those 20 pounds now for a 30-pound gain in six months?

How many times do you want to lose that 20 pounds?

I changed my mindset and decided to work the problem. Work. The. Problem. Remove as much emotion as possible. My body became a source of data. Nutrition and exercise were the variables I wanted to control. My results would be the side-effects of my consistent behaviors.

It's impossible to remove emotion from the act of eating entirely – it's social, it's security, etc. But to understand how I did what I did, you need to know how I changed my mindset. <u>I chose to look at nutrition as a problem-solving strategy</u>.

Problem: *I don't know how to feed myself properly.*

Solution: *I can fix it if I learn more. I need a teacher.*

My first nutrition coach, Kim, taught me how to measure and log food. She taught me how to use an online program to track it. I wore a gadget that estimated my calorie burn 24/7. When I started, I only used two numbers, calories burned and calories eaten, to gradually lose weight. I naturally gravitated towards more vegetables because you can eat more of those foods because they are less calorie-dense. Along the way, many myths were busted. Many lessons were learned.

If I could start-over, I would have done it a little differently. I will tell you how I would start now, knowing what I know now. But I started where I was, using what I knew at the time. Acting always works better than over-thinking and waiting.

Some lessons took longer to learn. I regret being a clean-eating-zealot-jerk who annoyed her friends. Sadly, I had to go through that phase to get to a place of balance that works for me now. Regardless of how poorly I handled it socially, my body responded well to the "clean" nutrition after decades of not getting enough micronutrients. Whole foods are still the foundation of my meals.

Over time, I learned how important flexibility of food choices are to sustainable program. Honestly, I hate to call it a "program". I eat to support my goals. Sometimes, I eat to be social. I love ice cream and have some every day except for when I'm close to a competition. It's not a treat. It's not a cheat. It's a food I like so I eat it. I've learned that less nutritious foods have an important purpose in my life. The provide psychological balance.

In this chapter, I'm sharing my personal experience and lessons I've learned. Before you make any changes to your own nutrition, please do your research and talk to your personal physician.

Where to Start? Establish Balance.

Every time I started a new "plan", I bought a lot of groceries!! And it didn't work. So, what did I learn? Don't replace all the foods you like. When it's time to make changes, make small ones. I know when you're motivated, the first thing that might happen is a trip to the grocery store to buy ALL the "heathy" foods.

That's <u>not</u> the first thing I would do now. Think about it – has that worked before? Or did you fall back into your old nutrition habits after a couple of weeks?

The first thing I would do now is to find the sweet spot where calories consumed during the day equals calories burned in a day. And it's better if you do that eating the foods you have been eating. (Trust me – the changes are coming, but not all at once.)

You need to find out how many calories <u>you</u> (not a generic human *like* you, but YOU) have to consume to maintain your weight at your <u>current</u> activity level. (Also, not adding activity just yet. It's coming.) Once you have that number, you can start adjusting variables like intake and activity to work towards your goal intelligently.

There are gadgets you can wear that will give you an estimate of your calorie burn. There are online calculators that you can use, too. But there are many variables that will adjust how your individual metabolism works. What you are really looking for is the number of calories you can eat that will keep your body weight fairly stable over time.

There is a straightforward, no-frills way to find that number. Track your intake and use a bathroom scale.

Logging Food is a Non-Negotiable (At First)

There is a learning curve to tracking food, but you've got to do it to get that calorie intake number. If you are using an online food tracker, enter your food as you eat it for a typical day. If possible, use a digital scale and measure your chosen portions in grams. Do that for everything you eat and include beverages that have calories.

Gather More Data

The next step is to add another data point – scale weight. I wanted to start losing weight right away, so this would feel counter-intuitive to me. But knowing what I know now, I would need this number to learn how to control intake and activity to make permanent fat-loss happen. I should have learned how to maintain my weight for a few weeks in the beginning.

When you have a good handle on tracking food, start weighing yourself daily. The goal is to keep that weight the same, plus or minus a couple of pounds over a couple of weeks. If you know you are accurately tracking food, and the scale weight at the end of a couple of weeks is about the same as it was on the first day, then you have found a good estimate for your personalized maintenance calorie intake number.

If you've had a history of dieting and regaining, it's possible that your body has adapted to lower calories and stores fat when you eat what you feel is a "normal" number of calories. That can be an adaptation to repeated dieting, but it can also be a symptom of a medical issue.

See your doctor first and tell them what is going on. They will know what to check and will advise you on how they want you to proceed.

After getting your doctor's approval, you may want to consider working with a nutrition coach to help you in the initial stages of your transformation. Nutrition coaches and trainers cannot diagnose or prescribe diets to treat medical conditions, so that's why you need to visit a physician first. Once a medical condition has been ruled out, a knowledgeable, science-based coach can help you, but it will take time. Remember – this is the LAST time you are starting over, so do it right!

Got Data! Now What?

Every person's body is different, so it would be irresponsible of me to give you an exact procedure about how to create the changes you want to see in your mirror or on your scale. I have no idea who is reading this and the variability between humans makes any "cookie-cutter" approach only effective for the small percentage of people who will respond well to that method. What I will do, is offer some general suggestions on how to get started based on what I've learned and my experience.

1) Do research! Learn for yourself why your body needs protein, carbs, and fats. Look for independent resources that are summaries of research and not selling a product. Despite what some "named" diets will tell you, you need all three macronutrients for optimal health. It's a misconception that different people will have the same results from those "named" diets that are low in a certain macronutrient. Those diets work for anyone who responds well to that particular combination. The people who don't get those results may think it's about their willpower, but it's highly likely that their body chemistry works better with a different combination of macronutrients. A good nutrition coach will help you individualize a combination of macros based on your goals and activity, while keeping your energy and moods as stable as possible. The more you learn about the science, the more likely you are to create a sustainable approach to nutritional self-care.

2) Find the macronutrient numbers on your food tracker – protein, carbohydrates, and fats. Research how to set your protein grams. Because I lift, I usually set mine to be equal to my body weight. For example, if I weigh 150 pounds, my protein intake would be about 150 grams on my daily tracker. If I've allowed my body fat to go up a bit, I won't increase protein to be scale weight, but still keep it around 150 grams. I keep protein intake fixed each day.

3) To lose weight safely, create a calorie deficit by reducing your intake of carbs, fats or both. Which one you cut is personal preference based on how you feel and the foods you like. The size of the deficits depends on the person and the goal, but it is suggested to keep that deficit as low as possible to see a <u>gradual</u> weight loss at the end of week. If you start out with a high deficit, you won't have any room later to increase it when your metabolism adapts and weight loss stalls. The goal is to trigger a gradual fat loss with a caloric deficit. It will take time, you'll have to be patient, but it is effective and likely to be sustainable.

4) Train with weights. The physical adaptations to lifting benefit fat loss. To change the shape of your body, you need to lift. Back in chapter 1, I described all the medical benefits I got from lifting.

Reflecting on what I did when I started, I think I made two mistakes. I did not pay attention to protein and I did not lift. I waited a year to start lifting. During that first year, my weight loss reversed, and I started gaining fat back while still in a calorie deficit. My only exercise was cardio.

Please know that no matter how you start, it won't be done perfectly and that's ok. Consistency is more important than perfection. What tends to frustrate people is that their results are never linear or predictable. That's normal. This is a marathon, not a sprint! It does work over time. Hang on to that thought when you're feeling like it's not working today. Or this week.

You will need to have a few refeeds along the way. May seem counter-intuitive, but it works. A refeed is when you bring your calories up to maintenance for a day. This is not a "cheat day". If you're not restricting your food choices and are eating foods you like, you probably won't feel too deprived. Just increase portion sizes or add in something to bring those calories up to maintenance. Do this once a week or once every two weeks.

If you've been consistent for a few months and weight loss has stalled, a diet break for a week is probably needed. Give your body a break. Let it rest for a few days. When you start again, you should see things getting back on track quickly. You can even plan these diet breaks to happen when there are social events scheduled.

What Happens If You Go Off the Rails?

It will happen. It happens to all of us and that's ok. **What hurts you more than the extra food is how you talk to yourself about screwing up.** You don't need to be perfect to make this work. It's probably better that you aren't. Learn to bounce back and not quit! This isn't an all-or-nothing process. Consistency matters and being consistent over time is going to get you to your goal.

Call it a "refeed" and get back on the program as soon as you can. If you can't log for some reason, eat what you usually eat. If you can't eat what you usually eat, keep portion sizes under control. Own that you <u>do</u> control what happens here. When things go sideways, grab the steering wheel and get yourself back on the road.

If you approach your nutrition as a component of self-care, if you pay attention to how you are feeling and how well you recover from workouts, and if you commit to keeping your mind open, you will learn about yourself while you learn more about nutrition. Don't lose your balance by jumping around from program to program just because other people swear by it. This isn't about a short-term goal – this is about learning to care for yourself and undo years of neglect.

Chapter 8 Notes

Eating 101

Chapter 9

Lifting – How Do I Start?

"The heart of the discerning acquires knowledge,
for the ears of the wise seek it out."
Proverbs 18:15

"Do the best you can until you know better. Then when you
know better, do better."
Maya Angelou

> *The information in this chapter is meant to supplement, not replace, proper personal training in weightlifting. Like any form of exercise, strength training poses some inherent risk. The author and publisher advise readers to take full responsibility for their safety and know their limits. Do not take risks beyond your level of experience, aptitude, training, and comfort level.*

The Maya Angelou quote above describes my evolution as a lifter perfectly. I can't stress enough how important it is just to start. Start imperfectly. You're a newb – embrace it. Yes, you're going to feel awkward. And yes, you're going to look a bit awkward. But it's not the first time you've started something and didn't really know what you were doing. If you don't start and commit to learning this skill, you'll never become more accomplished. Not many people approach lifting as a skill - that's a mistake.

Let's talk about the elephant in the room before going on. Someone reading this right now wants to learn how to lift but is scared. You might fear looking stupid. You might be scared that other people in the gym will judge you or laugh at you because you are weak, fat, too old, or don't belong there. I know _exactly_ how much courage it takes to just walk into a gym if you don't feel like you belong there. I _know_.

Once at the gym, you may feel like you must stick to cardio or go into a side room and do your own thing for a while. That's ok. But if you haven't started lifting yet because you don't know how, my suggestion is that you muster up your courage, change your paradigm about doing this yourself, and work with a trainer for a month or two. Make it work.

Personally, I rationalized paying for training as "getting help" just like I "got help" from doctors with my high blood pressure. But that's me and I was able to make it work. I know each person must find their own path.

Status: Beginner

My best advice is to get clearance from your doctor to start a lifting program first, then work with a personal trainer. I worked with a trainer because I knew I needed help and didn't want to waste my time learning the wrong things. If you are new to this activity, you need help, too. If I need a filling, I don't do that myself either – I go to the dentist. My first trainer did an assessment on my conditioning, muscle imbalances, flexibility and general balance. I was a mess. The first few months were dedicated to functional work.

As a beginner, your focus needs to be on the following:

- Establish the habit of exercise.

- Build core strength. "Core" is not just abdominals. Your core includes deep muscles that are your foundation and not visible. They surround your spine. Also, think about bringing up the functionality of all big muscle groups from a deconditioned state. Your tendons and ligaments are also not ready to handle lifting just yet. People forget about training connective tissues, but if you experience an injury at some point, it will likely be a connective tissue strain or tear. Muscles can handle more stress than connective tissues.

- Commit to using proper form at all times! If your trainer is not analyzing your form, ask them to do that. If they still don't pay attention, get a new trainer. You should also do your own research. Watch videos online for exercises you know you are going to do.

- Avoid using momentum when lifting. If you need to swing it to move it, it's too heavy. Control the movement and focus on the muscle you are working. For example, if you're doing an exercise to work triceps, but feel it in your shoulders, check your form and/or lower the weight.

Because there are things you need to pay attention to as you are moving a weight through space – form, muscles worked, proper load, etc. – this is why I want you to think of lifting as a

SKILL that needs to be practiced. You will become a better lifter, have better results, and be able to do it safely for the rest of your life if you focus on improving your technical skills.

I worked on functional training with my trainer for months. The day my trainer let me work with a barbell was a happy one! That's when I started to feel like this bodybuilding thing might become a reality.

If you are designing your own program, you don't need to start with anything complicated. Luckily, new lifters will make dramatic progress by just starting and lifting consistently. Begin with a whole-body routine done three times a week for a couple of months. Once you have picked exercises you like to do, exercises that feel comfortable for your personal body-geometry, stick to that routine for a couple of months before you think about changing things up. You need to allow yourself time to get stronger and progress in the same movements.

Keep a Log

You will need to keep track of your lifting progress. Keep this part simple. There are phone apps that will do it, but in the beginning, there is so much to learn while establishing this new habit, that I suggest you go "old school" and use a notebook and a pen.

Here is how you can record your work. If you did 1 set of 8 repetitions with 50 pounds on the leg press machine, write:

Leg Press: 1 x 8 x 50

For an absolute beginner in the gym who is not working with a trainer, use the machines at first for lifting. Machines will keep you in proper form. Always start with the biggest muscle groups first before you work smaller ones. For example, do chest presses and back pulldowns before arms. Do exercises that work more than one muscle group before doing isolation movements. For instance, do leg presses before leg extensions or leg curls. Do core strengthening and stabilizing exercises like planks at the end of your workout.

Beginner: Basic Workout Blueprint

1) Warm up. I like to walk for a few minutes on the treadmill. Then I will do light activation movements with

elastic bands to activate the muscle groups I'm going to use. Some people like to do flexibility (also called mobility) work during their warm ups. Watch some videos online about warming up. Don't skip this part – ever.

2) Do one set of one exercise for each muscle group, larger muscle groups before smaller ones. Always do a couple of warm-up sets with no weight or very light weight. This will allow you to focus on form before there is a load. It also allows you to check on your connective tissues to make sure you're able to do the movement in full range of motion. When doing working sets, choose a weight that allows you to complete 8 to 12 repetitions <u>with proper form</u>. The last few reps should feel harder, but not so heavy that you lose form.

    a. Large Muscle Groups: chest, back, quadriceps, hamstrings

    b. Smaller Muscle Groups: shoulders, arms, calves

3) Do core work. Planks and choose another abdominal exercise if you want. But don't skip planks. They are the best exercise for developing your deep core muscles.

4) Cooldown. This is a good time to stretch.

What About Pain?

It's important to learn the difference between pain that is a normal part of lifting or pain due to a possible injury. If you're at the end of a set and it burns a little, that's normal. If it feels like something in your joint – **STOP**. If it is a sharp pain – **STOP**. If you're not sure – **STOP**. With lifting, it is better to back off. Don't go "beast mode" – you could push a mild strain into a more serious injury. Instead, think "live to fight another day".

Most pain you may experience from lifting will happen the next day or a couple days after a lift. It's called DOMS (Delayed Onset Muscle Soreness). You probably know what this feels like already from that time you moved a lot of boxes or did a lot of yard work. It's normal.

DOMS may not always happen and it doesn't have to happen for you to get stronger or grow muscle. When you lift, you are making tiny tears in the tissue. When they heal, you will be stronger. Some pain is part of this and lifters learn to tell the difference between "normal" pain and a possible injury. (The irony is that most lifters don't get hurt in the gym. They get hurt doing something around the house or at work.)

Why do you need to lift? If you don't do any resistance training, you're going to lose muscle and bone mass as you age. Without muscle and solid bones, a simple fall can be traumatic. Strength training, done mindfully, will prevent injuries in daily life.

Status: Intermediate

Most people will be beginners for a few months if consistent. It has more to do with your development and capacity than with time. When your base strength is enough so that you can handle barbells, it's time to change up the program to continue your progress. Again – don't change it too frequently or else you will not continue to progress!

If you were working with a trainer, but no longer need them to be with you when you lift, they might agree to write a program for you. Or, you could work with an online coach, which is usually a more affordable option. Work with people who stay current with exercise science and are willing to customize a program for you and your goals. Most people who lift for general fitness will be able to reach their goals as intermediate lifters. Athletes who want to compete in a physique or strength sport, might want to consider having a science-based prep coach or strength coach do their programming.

Program Designs to Research

If you're interested in designing your own program, I'm going to mention only a few approaches of the dozens out there. I want to give you a few ideas about where to start your research. I won't get into too much detail about each design. For most people who are not competitors, any of these variations will work. Honestly, most long-time lifters will use all of them at some point. You may find one that works better with your life or how you feel when you train. Personally, I like upper/lower splits. But I know people who like the push/pull split. Nothing is carved in stone. You can adjust things to make it work for you.

One Body Part a Day (5-Day Split)

With this approach, each major muscle group has its own workout and it's done once a week. This is an "old school" approach and is popular because that's how lifters used to organize their programs back in the day. If you are a beginner transitioning to an intermediate lifter, it's a good place to start as you incorporate more free weights into your program. You will still see progress. Working a body part once a week allows for more time to recover, too.

Upper / Lower (2-Day Split)

With this design, you do your upper body movements one day and your lower body movements the next day. A variation is to make this a 3-day split with arms and calves on the third day. Abs can be done on either day. The upper/lower split is my favorite. I've varied how I organized it in my week. Sometimes I've lifted for two days and rested the third day. I've also done it where I've lifted every-other day.

Push / Pull (2-Day Split)

With this design, you organize your main lifts based on the type of movement. Dumbbell rows are a pull-movement. Bench press is a push-movement. The thinking behind push/pull organization is that it reduces stress on the same muscle groups during the week. For example, if you worked chest yesterday and triceps today, you're working triceps twice in two days because they are a "pushing" muscle and are used when you bench press. Which means, you also worked the connective tissues twice in two days, which may not be desirable.

What about Cardio?

Cardio? Do you mean lifting weights faster? (Joking.) I don't hate cardio, but for a bodybuilder, it's a tool. When I'm in a building phase, I don't do as much because my goal is to gain weight – ideally muscle, but the fat comes along with it. I don't cut cardio out entirely. I need a little cardio for stress management and mood regulation. My main cardio activity is walking because I'm a dog-mom. Dogs need to be walked and don't seem to care about my bodybuilding program. Even when in contest prep, walking is my primary cardio activity.

There is a LOT of information out there about cardio. Most of it makes it seem too complicated. Choose what you like, what won't stress your knees and feet too much, and what you will be willing to do.

The reason it's just a tool for a lifter is that the main reason we look the way we look is a result of lifting. The body adapts to its training. If your training program is based on an endurance activity like running, you will look like a runner. If your training program is designed to prepare you for a strongman competition, you will look like a strongman competitor.

If your goal is to build muscle, keep cardio and lifting separate if possible. Wear and tear on connective tissues from a cardio session before lifting can put the lifter at risk for injury. Also, any nutrients you have in your system need to be used for energy and recovery from lifting. You do not want to divert those resources to supply energy for the cardio session.

If you're still thinking about starting a lifting program, it's time to make the decision and start. At risk of sounding repetitive – how you start doesn't matter as much as just getting started. As you learn more, you'll make changes. Every lifter was a beginner.

Chapter 9 Notes

Lifting – How Do I Start?

Chapter 10

Ten Tips to Start Your Transformation

"She is clothed with strength and dignity, and she laughs
without fear of the future."
Proverbs 31:25

"Go confidently in the direction of your dreams! Live the life
you've imagined. As you simplify your life, the laws of the
universe will be simpler."
Henry David Thoreau

Are you ready to start your own sustainable transformation? I've consolidated the advice I've given in this book into these 10 tips to help you see the big picture as you make decisions and plans.

Tip 1: Collect current data about your food intake.

Start with an honest inventory of what and how much you're eating now. Eat normally, but log it for a full week, at least. Better if you can make it a habit. You will need to measure and weigh food to log it accurately. Get a digital scale to make this chore easier. I've used a digital scale every day since I started, and I've never used an expensive one. Use an online food log to have access to an extensive database. It takes a little time to learn to do log efficiently, but if you're using an online tracker, it becomes a matter of clicking frequent foods instead of searching.

Tip 2: Come up with a reasonable estimate of how many calories you burn in a 24-hour period.

I remember that "ah-ha" moment when I realized that I'm burning calories all the time, not just when I exercise. There are calculators online that will give a very rough estimate, but they cannot be accurate. If you have a history of repeated dieting, your metabolism may have been changed a bit, so the online formulas will return a number that is too high for you. If you can make an investment, there are gadgets that you wear that will give better estimates based on your personal activity over the entire day. I do like my gadget! However, to start, you only need that maintenance number of calorie intake that keeps your weight stable.

Tip 3: Make a food plan based on what you do now.

There is a minimum number of calories you need to eat for general health. One technique to estimate the number of calories a person needs to *maintain* their weight is to take 15 times (body weight in pounds). For example, a person who weighs 150 pounds, theoretically will maintain their weight with 15 x 150 = 2,250 calorie intake a day. But honestly, that number is another one that needs to be individualized based on a person's history with dieting and current lifestyle. If that same 150-pound person learns through tracking and checking scale weight, that she maintains her weight with an intake of 1500 calories, jumping up to 2,250 will cause a weight gain.

I'm not saying the math doesn't work. What I am saying, is that <u>your</u> unique formula based on your genetics and dieting history probably isn't going to be something you will find online. You need to track your intake data and compare it with scale weight averages over a week or two to figure out what is true for you. You are looking to <u>balance intake with scale weight over time</u> to find your maintenance calorie number.

To lose fat safely, create a moderate calorie deficit between what you eat and what you burn in a 24-hour period. How much of a deficit? This depends on the person's situation. If someone's metabolism is healthy, I'd suggest a deficit of 300 to 800 calories. But if a person is maintaining their weight on a calorie intake that doesn't have enough "cushion" to create a deficit, it's healthier to post-pone a fat-loss phase and work with someone to improve the metabolism first. Otherwise, the weight will come back – and bring friends.

It is important to get your own baseline data about maintenance calories before you make any changes in your intake or activity. You want to make small changes at first, so you can keep adjusting later when your progress stalls.

Tip 4: Make food substitutions gradually.

It is not practical for most people to completely replace everything in the kitchen. Food prep may be a new routine that will change how you spend your time. At first, you'll be inefficient with your time as you work things out. And it is hard to establish a new habit. That's OK. Hard doesn't mean impossible. It does get easier.

Tip 5: Train with weights.

It's not a hard sell to tell someone they need to lift to build muscle. But many people just want to lose weight – which really means *fat-loss*. A cardio-only program is not optimal if the goal is to change body composition. There are several reasons why resistance training needs to be part of a program for fat loss. Resistance training preserves muscle and builds bone mass. To change the appearance of the body, the muscles need to be developed.

Even if lifting isn't your favorite thing to do, think of it as self-care and figure out how to make it part of your week. Your body is made up of bones, muscles, tendons, and ligaments that need to be used for optimum health.

Tip 6: Don't overdo cardio.

There is an abundance of science and opinions out there about cardio. Do your research, but also pay attention to how you feel. My body responds to long sessions of cardio by elevating cortisol levels. Cortisol is a hormone similar to adrenaline. I believe I've had a cortisol problem for a long time and it contributed to anxiety, weight gain, and my health decline. When my cortisol levels are up, I feel very anxious and I have trouble falling asleep. It's an unpleasant feeling.

Tip 7: Sleep.

The body needs to rest to recover from the stress of the day. When you add exercise and a moderate calorie restriction, there will be more stress on the body. Lack of sleep will elevate cortisol levels, too.

Tip 8: Drink water.

The body uses water to process nutrients, lubricate joints, maintain healthy blood pressure – well, just about everything. If you research this topic online, you'll get a lot of different recommendations. The general rule of thumb is about a half-gallon a day. Personally, I feel better with a gallon. As in all things, results will vary because we aren't all the same, we aren't all living in the same climate, aren't all eating the same foods, etc. Again – pay attention to how you're feeling and adapt.

Tip 9: Keep it simple.

Avoid the urge to over-plan, despite all the information I've just thrown at you. Your program does not have to be perfect. As you learn more, you'll adjust things. You have to <u>move</u>, so pick your favorite activity for exercise so you'll be more inclined to do it. You do need to consume more whole foods for the nutrients, but don't completely deprive yourself of things you enjoy. ***This isn't a program***. This is how you are going to live now, so it needs to be realistic and sustainable.

Tip 10: Be Patient.

Permanent changes happen slowly. You are changing your life one cell at a time. It's a habit to feel impatient, especially when looking at someone's transformation picture because the eye just goes back forth between the two versions of that person. But note the dates. Took me <u>three years</u> to get from "before" to the first "after" picture in 2012. What helped me when I felt impatient, when things seem to be stalled, was to remind myself that this was the LAST time I was going to lose most of these fat pounds. My life was going to be different because I wouldn't stop practicing self-care ever again.

I didn't love this stuff at first. But I do now. I'm happier, excited to get up every day, and my life is likely to be longer because I decided to do this thing and not quit.

Chapter 10 Notes

Ten Tips to Start Your Transformation

Conclusion

Faith and Gratitude

"Don't be afraid, for I am with you.
Don't be discouraged, for I am your God.
I will strengthen you and help you.
I will hold you up with my victorious right hand."
Isaiah 41:10

Faith

My mother's unexpected death when I was 29 years old changed me. I was a single woman in Minneapolis, Minnesota only responsible for myself. My mother was handling my grandmother's estate at the time of her own death, so it fell to me to manage the affairs of both my mother and grandmother. The weekend before my mother's death, I was out clubbing with friends. A few days later, I watched my mother die, and the week after that, I was fired when I asked for a leave-of-absence so I could have a little time to figure out how to manage TWO estates alone while grieving. I had gone back to college to earn my teaching degree a few months before and was supposed to start final exams about 10 days later. Only one professor agreed to issue an incomplete. (I'll never forget her kindness and am still grateful for it.)

Prayer was part of my life when I was younger. I let it go. But I needed God to be back in my life if I had any chance of navigating what was ahead. This prayer went up while sitting in my car in a parking garage at my university when I drove back to take those final exams…

"I promise. I'll do the work.
Just point me in the right direction."

The second time that prayer went up was after the emergency room visit in 2009. I've had that conversation with God many times in recent years.

There have been several times when I wanted to get off this bodybuilding path because I was frustrated with the life lessons, crushed by the setbacks, or uncomfortable with the public attention. I'm sure I will continue to question why I'm doing all of this – especially now that I've made my life more "public" by writing this book.

But every time I question it, a reminder comes to get back on the path He put me on. Every. Single. Time. I'm not exaggerating. If I question it, a course correction comes. It's usually from a follower who found the courage to start self-care from finding my story posted somewhere online.

Prayer helps me stay positive and focused. My faith is personal, but it is important for me to share this with you because I would not have been able to what I've done without His help. He's always been there for me when it was just too much for me to do alone.

With Gratitude – Time for my "Thank You's"!

First and always - my husband Paul. You didn't sign up for any of this, wasn't sure about this "bodybuilding" thing at first but supported me anyway. Your advice and wisdom help me stay centered. Your love and encouragement mean everything to me.

To Kim, my first nutrition coach – thank you!!! Your patience, positivity, and support while teaching me how to feed myself properly made me believe this was possible.

To American Iron Gym – thank you for 'adopting' me when I was lost. The morning crew stepped up and filled in as my trainers when I still didn't know what I was doing. Thank you, Bob and Tammy! You have created a space for lifters that always inspires me every time I walk in.

To Dietrich – thank you for coaching me and holding my hand through my first two shows. I learned so much from you!

Hey Berto!! I'm so grateful for you! We are an unlikely coach/athlete team, aren't we? But it works. I've learned so much from you. You have taught me how to make a bodybuilding life healthy, balanced, and rooted in self-care. You consistently share your belief in my capacity to do this sport. I lean on you when I have doubts.

Finally – to my followers on the Facebook Lifting My Spirits page – THANK YOU! Many of you have been traveling with me since 2013. You've been there to offer encouragement and support. You've been there to do battle with trolls when that was necessary. You've shared your fears and successes with me, too. Those stories have kept me going when I wanted to quit. In my mind, we are a community and I am grateful for you!!

Dear Reader – thank you!! I'm a first-time author, so if you struggled a bit to get through this book, I apologize. My heart is in these pages, though. If anyone borrows a little courage to begin and sustain their own health-transformation, my goal for this book will have been achieved. If that's you, feel free to reach out and share your story with me. I'd love to hear from you! You can contact me at LiftingMySpirtitsBook@gmail.com.

If you enjoyed the book and found anything in it helpful, please consider leaving a review on Amazon. It helps others who have no idea who I am or why I'm writing a book to read your thoughts.

Thank you and God bless!

2008

2009

2012

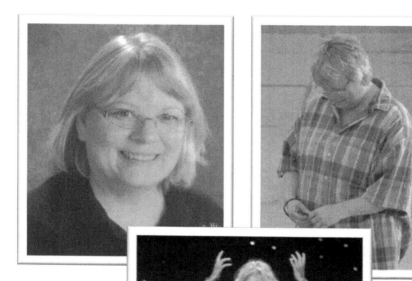

2015

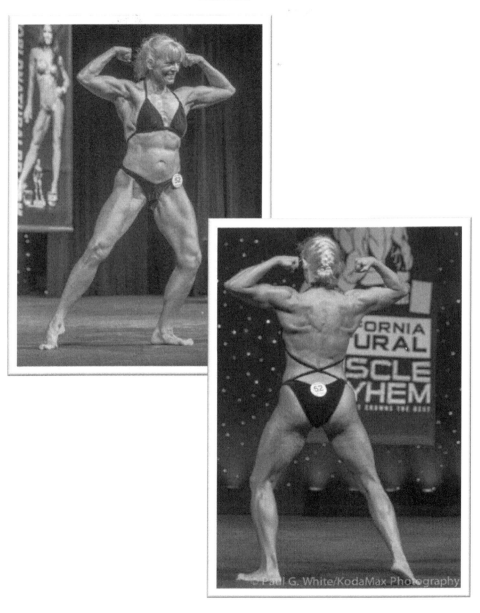

© Paul G. White/KodaMax Photography

2017

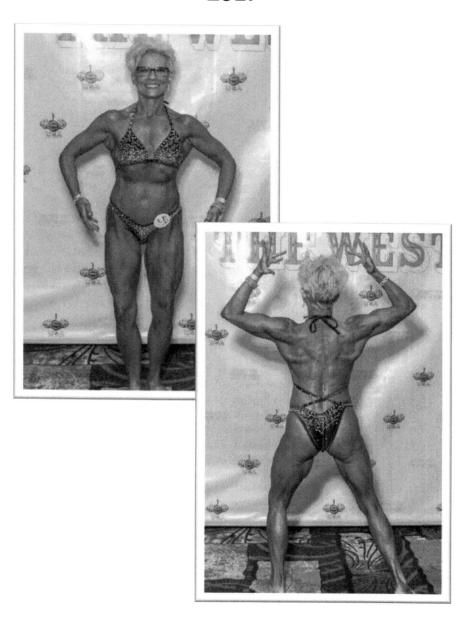

About the Author

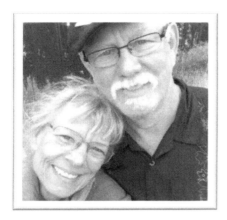

TAMMY WHITE is a wife and a retired high school math teacher. A health scare changed her perspective about aging and set her on a path to live differently. She always admired the female bodybuilders from the 1980's, so while her primary goal was to repair damage to her health from years of self-neglect, she set her "Big Scary Goal" to become a competitive bodybuilder by age 50. She has learned that the same science-based best-practices used to push her fat-loss to an extreme as a bodybuilder can help the general population reach their less-extreme goals. She is using her NASM Fitness Nutrition Specialist certification, her teaching skill set to empower while educating, combined with almost a decade of personal experience to help people from around the world as an online Nutritional Consultant and Accountability Coach.

Made in the USA
Columbia, SC
09 August 2019